The A to Z of Respiration

Introduction

This book is a referen: the
It is the 16th book in
A to Z website listed I
whether online or not
and I thank those of y
series. Believe me th
reached. I hope this i.

ort
d,
is
evel is

The A to Zs may be viewed on 3 sites –
www.amandasatoz.com and
http://www.aspenpharma.com.au/atlas/student.htm
http://www.aspenpharma.com.au
Feedback may be left at
mandasatoz@gmail.com

Acknowledgement

Thank you Aspen Australia for your support and assistance in this valuable project.

Dedication

To those who support this project and have done so for many years. To my friends and colleagues, many of whom work at Aspen. It is possible things are changing with respect to Anatomy - many medical and other healthcare students including nursing students have pushed for more anatomy in their courses. Indeed there is a push in the community for more understanding of the components and working of this wonderful machine - the human body - so I also dedicate this book to the wonderful human body.

How to use this book

The format of this A to Z book has been maintained.

The Common Terms (CT) section comments on a number of processes & pathologies in the respiratory system, while the Main Text (MT) is alphabeticalized as usual, & has 3 subsections: the Respiratory Cells, the Function & the Structures of the Respiratory System. The cross-referencing b/n the 2 sections & other A to Zs has been expanded, as requested via feedback comments. So as usual ***think of it and then find it*** is the motto ***of the A to Zs*** and continues to be the structure behind the book. Additional information may found in all the A to Zs but in particular *The A to Z of the*

Head & Neck Bones & Muscles, **The A to Z of Major Organs**, *The A to Z of the Brain & Cranial Nerves*, **The A to Z of the Heart**, & **The A to Z of the Digestive Tract**, and in some instances the reader is guided to these areas and other areas of interest via QR codes inserted strategically into this book. However as with all the A to Zs this book is complete unto itself.

Thank you
A. L. Neill
BSc MSc MBBS PhD FACBS

TABLE OF CONTENTS

The Cells of the Respiratory Tract

The Functions of the Respiratory System

The Structures of the Respiratory System

Abbreviations of the terms used in Respiration

A

a	artery
aa	anastomosis (ses)
AA	amino acid
AB	acid/base
Ab	antibody
ACTH	adrenocorticotropic hormone / adrenal cortical hormone
adj.	adjective
ADP	adenosine diphosphate
ADS	**anatomical dead space**
AF	air flow
Ag	antigen
AKA	also known as
alt.	alternative
ALTH	**acclimatization to hypoxia - long term**
AMP	adenosine monophosphate
ANS	autonomic nervous system
ant.	anterior
art	artery
AP	anterior – posterior
AQP	aquaporin
AR	**Airways resistance**
AS	Alternative Spelling, generally referring to the diff. b/n British & American spelling
ASTH	**acclimatization to hypoxia - short term**
ATP	adenosine triphosphate
a&v	artery and vein

B

b	bone
B	blood
BALT	**bronchus associated lymphoid tissue**
BB	basal bodies
bc	because
BGB	blood / gas / barrier
BM	basement membrane / basal lamina / terminal lamina / plasma lamina
b/n	between

bn	bone
BP	blood pressure
br	branch
BS	Blood Supply

C

cAMP	yclic AMP
cart	cartilage
CC	costal cartilage
CCF	congestive heart failure
c.f.	compared to
CF	cystic fibrosis
CFA	cryptogenic fibrosing alveolitis
CM	cellular membrane / plasma membrane
CMV	controlled mechanical ventilation
CMV	cytomegalovirus
CNS	central nervous system
COAD	***chronic obstructive airway disease***
COLD	***chronic obstructive lung disease***
COPD	***chronic obstructive pulmonary disease***
CP	cervical plexus
CPAP	**continuous positive airway pressure**
collat.	collateral
Cr	cranial
CT	connective tissue / computed tomography
CT	common terms section of this book ($\neq$ MT)
CXR	chest Xray

D

DNA	deoxyribonucleic acid
DOPA	dihydroxyphenylalanine
DT	digestive tract
diff.	difference(s)
dist.	distal
DM	dura mater
DT	digestive tract

E

E	energy
e.g.	example
EAM	external acoustic meatus
EC	extracellular (outside the cell)
ECF	extracellular fluid
ER	endoplasmic reticulum
ext.	extensor (as in muscle to extend across a joint)

F

FRC	Functional Residual Capacity
FVC	Forced Vital Capacity

G

GA	Golgi apparatus
gld	gland
Gk.	Greek
GM	grey matter
GN	Golgi network
grp	group

H

H	hormone
Hb	haemoglobin
H&E	haematoxylin & eosin
Hg	haemorrhage
HP	high pressure / high power - wrt magnification

I

IAM	internal acoustic meatus
IC	**intercostal**
IC	intracellular (inside the cell)
ICS	**intercostal space**
IF	inflammation
ImR	immune response
inf	inferior
In	infection
IR	inflammatory response
IVC	inferior vena cava
Iy	injury

J

JC	junctional complex
jt(s)	joints = articulations

L

l	lymphatic
lig	ligament
L	lumbar / left
LA	**lower airways**
LB	lamellar bodies
lig	ligament
LP	lamina propria / lateral process
LP	low power - wrt magnification
LRT	**lower respiratory tract**
LT	lymphoid tissue
Lt.	Latin
LUQ	left upper quadrant
LV	left ventricle/ lung volume

M

m	muscle
med.	medial
mem	membrane
mito	mitochondrion (a)
MM	mucus membrane
mRNA	messenger RNA
MT	main text of this book ($\neq$ CT)
mv	microvillus(i)

N

N(s)	nerve(s)
NAD	normal (size, shape)
NAD	no abnormality detected
NM	nuclear membrane / nucleolemma
NR	nerve root origin
NRAM	non-respiratory air movement
NS	nerve supply / nervous system
NT	nervous tissue
nv	neurovascular bundle

O

O	origin
OSA	obstructive sleep apnea

P

pl.	plural
ParaNS	parasympathetic nervous system
PDS	**physiological dead space**
PN	peripheral nerve
PND	**posterior nasal drip**
post.	posterior
proc.	process
prox.	proximal
PSCCE	pseudo-stratified columnar ciliated epithelium

Q

Q	perfusion

R

R	right / resistance
R&L	right and left
REM	rapid eye movement
RNA	ribonucleic acid
rRNA	ribosomal RNA
RT	respiratory tract
RUQ	right upper quadrant
RV	right ventricle (of the heart)
RZ	**respiratory zone**

S

SA	surface area
SC	spinal cord
sing.	singular
SN	spinal nerve
SP	surfactant proteins
SS	signs & symptoms
St	surface tension
subcut.	subcutaneous (just under the skin)
sup	superior

| supf | superficial |
| SymNS | sympathetic nervous system |

T

T	thoracic / thorax / tissue
TJ	tight junctional complexes
TNF	tumour necrosis factor
tRNA	transfer RNA / transport RNA
TRU	**terminal respiratory unit**
TZ	**transport zone**

U

UA	**upper airways**
UL	upper limb / arm
URT	**upper respiratory tract**

V

V	vein / vertebra
V	ventilation
v	very
VB	vertebral body
VC	vocal cord / vertebral column / vital capacity
VF	vocal fold
V/Q	**ventilation / perfusion ratio**
vv	visa versa

W

WM	white matter
w/n	within
w/o	without
wrt	with respect to

Z

| ZA | zonula adherens |
| ZO | zonula occludens / tight junction |

SYMBOLS

| & | and |
| ∩ | intersection with |

Common terms used to describe Breathing, Smelling & Respiration

Pronunciation Key & Colour Guide

Most terms are listed in black

Pathological terms are in green

Prefixes and Suffixes are in blue

Specific respiratory definitions are listed separately in indigo

The pronunciation guide to words in this section are in bold red lettering

Stressed syllables are in **CAPITAL LETTERS**

Vowel sounds are pronounced as indicated below

A	May	ay
	map	a
	mark	ah
E	Me	ee
	met	e
	term	ur
I	eye / sight	ï
	tin	i
O	go	oh
	mother	uh
	mop	o
	more	or
	boy	oi
	lose	oo
	nook	oe
	loose	ou
U	blue	ou
	cute	ew
	cut	uh
Y	family	ee
	myth	i
	eye	ï

Common Terms used in Respiration

A

a- without, lack of, no

α-antitrypsin: any of a grp of glycoproteins migrating in the α region on serum electrophoresis & capable of inhibiting trypsin & other proteolytic enzymes

ab– away from , negative

Abdomen: *Lt. abdomen = the belly,* the part of the trunk b/n thorax & the perineum,

Abduction: *Lt. ab = from, & ductum = led,* hence, movement from; verb - abduct. (≠ Adduction)

Aberrant: *Lt. ab = from, and errare = to wander,* hence, deviating from normal.

Abscess (AB-sess): *Lt: abscessus = pus* localized collection of pus mainly PMNs accumulated as a defence mechanism against the presence of infective material &/or FBs

Absorption (ab-SORB-shun): the passage of material, from a lumen of an organ into another body space, T or cell

ac- toward, near to, addition to

Accessory: *Lt. accessum = added,* hence, supplementary.

Acetylcholine (a-set-tĭl KOHL-een): a neurotransmitter produced by the ParaNs

Acidaemia: an abnormally low (acidic) pH of the B (≠ Alkalaemia)

Acidosis: a disturbance of the AB in the body - towards the acid (≠ Alkalosis)

Acini (AS-ee-nee): clusters of cells which face a lumen may be part of an exocrine gland or involved in GE, beginning with respiratory bronchioles & ending with alveoli . *sing. acinus (AS-een-us) adj. acinar*

acro- extremity

Actin (AK-tin): *Gk: actinos* – ray the contractile protein that makes up the major portion of thin filaments in muscle fibers, & is one of the filamentous components in cilia *see also Cilia.*

acu- sudden, sharp , severe

Acute (AK-yewt): *Gk: acu- acus = needle* sharp, sudden onset + short course pathological process – used to describe any condition which starts suddenly & is of short duration; may be associated with a sharp needle-like pain of relatively short duration, although the 2 separate processes may co-exist, c.f. acute-on-chronic - describes a flare up of a chronic disease. (≠ Chronic)

ad- near, toward

Adam's apple AKA Laryngeal cartilage AKA Thyroid cartilage *see MT Larynx*

Additus: *Lt. = entrance, opening*

Adduction: *Lt. ad = to, & ductum = led*, hence, movement towards; *verb - adduct.* (≠ Abduction)

aden- gland

Adenoids AKA Palatine tonsils: *Gk. aden = a gland, eidos = shape or form*. groups of LNs at the back of the nose N which may swell S & block both the nose & the eustachian tubes causing breathing, hearing & speech difficulties particularly in young children, who proportionately have larger tonsils & smaller noses than adults

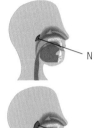

Adhesion: *Lt. ad = to, & haesus = stuck*

–aemia AS -emia pertaining to B, generally RBCs

Aerosol: a suspension in the air or other gaseous medium of minute solid &/or liquid particles

Afferent: coming towards e.g. Ns coming into the Brain - afferent Ns are sensory Ns ≠ **Efferent**

Agglutination: the process of things sticking together as in Ag/Ab complexes & RBCs

Airways Resistance (AR): the R to flow of gas presented in the airways of the lungs analogous to the R to current in an electrical wire

Alkalaemia: an abnormally high (alkalinic) pH of the B (≠ **Acidaemia**)

Alkalosis: a disturbance of the AB in the body - towards the alkaline - arterial pH > 7.45 (≠ **Acidosis**)

Allergen Ag: a substance (usually an Ag) which causes a vigorous ImR i.e. an allergic reaction

Allergic rhinitis AKA Hayfever: IF of the nose/nasal passages due to an overreaction of the ImR. Swollen nasal mucosa leads to a blocked nose & tear ducts. Nasal secretions ↑ as well as nasal irritation, causing: coughing, sneezing, crying & swelling.

Allergy: an overreaction of the immune system to a stimulus that otherwise would not be harmful tens to involve the epithelium of the RT, DT &/or skin, *adj allergic see also Anaphylaxis, Atopy allergic rhinitis*

Alveolar dead space the region of the alveoli that is ventilated (V) but not perfused (Q), or underperfused V/Q >1. This varies & should be small in healthy subjects. It is part of the physiological dead space.

Alveolar gas equation: defines the relationship b/n alveolar [gas], the inspired [gas] & the expired [gas] & alveolar ventilation

Alveolar sac: the last generation of air passages in the lungs; blind ended alveolar ducts. There are equal numbers of sacs & ducts - both involved in GE.

Alveolus: air filled cavity e.g. in the lung the small sacs in the GE region of the lungs *adj - alveolar*; (as in air filled bone in the Maxilla) *pl - alveoli*

ambi- both, about, around

amin(o)- an organic substance containing nitrogen

an- without, lack of, not

an(a)- up, back, again, excessive

Anaemia AS Anemia: *w/o blood* hence lack of RBCs

Anaphylaxis: severe allergic reaction

Anatomical dead space (ADS): air reaching the alveoli which does not take place in the GE e.g. from the nose & mouth to the terminal bronchioles

angio- (ANJ-ee-oh) to do with BVs

Anions: negatively charged atoms or radicals e.g. Cl-, OH-

anomalo- uneven, irregular

Anoxia (AN-oks-see-yuh): lack of oxygen in the B or Ts

ante- (AN-tee) before

Antenatal: *Lt. ante = before, & nato = birth* hence before the birth

Anterior (ant.) (ant-TEE-re-or): *Lt. ante = in front (in place or time).* a directional term describing the location of a part being toward the front or near side relative to another part.

antero- anterior, forward

anti- against, combating

Antibody (Ab) / Antigen (Ag): proteins involved in the immune system – antibodies *Abs* are produced by the body in reaction to antigens *Ags* proteins or materials found on the surface of FBs introduced to the body forming the **Ab/Ag** complex

Antitussive: an intervention aimed at reducing the cough

ap- toward , near to

ap- away from derived from, separation

Aperture (AP-ert-yew-er): an opening or space b/n bones or w/n a bone.

Apex (AY-pex): the extremity of a conical or pyramidal structure. The apex of the lung is the top of the lung & it extends above the thoracic outlet & hence is not protected by the ribs

Apnoea (AP-nee-ya): *Lt. a = without, & pneo = breath* lack of breathing *see also MT - sleep apnea*

Apnoeustic: prolonged breath holding in inspiration

Apoptysis (AP-pop- te-sis): *Gk aptos = to drop out* describes pockets of dead or dying cells - found in all organs wedged b/n healthy cells so it is thought to be a physiological phenomenon of normal aging or cellular weeding out

Appendicular: refers to the appendices of the axial i.e. in the skeleton, the arms & legs which hang from the axial skeleton; this also includes the pectoral & pelvic girdles (not the Sacrum) *noun appendix* as in the vermiform appendix

Aquaporins: protein group in the CM to facilitate the passage of water - particularly in secretions & larger flow. Water channels (wc) can be seen in the structure of the protein, when viewed from the correct orientation

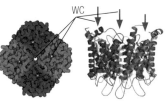

Arbor: *Gk treelike branches – arborizing*, branching

Arytenoid: ladle or pitcher wrt respiratory system - the arytenoid cartilages(1) move in & out like ladle with changing sounds & are attached to the Cricoid cartilage(2), which also

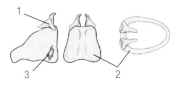

articulates with the thyroid cartilage's inferior horn via its side facet(3) *see also Cricoid, MT Larynx*

asthen- weak, weakness

Aspiration: the act of drawing foreign material into the lungs. This may occur with vomitus, which means in the pharynx & then is inhaled (mainly into the R lung).

Asthma: an airway disease with SS due to reversible intermittent airway obstruction. There is often an infiltrate of eosinophils, & an association with allergic diseases

Atelectasis (AT-e-lek-TAY-sis): *Gk ateles- incomplete , ektasis – opening* hence incomplete opening of the lungs/or collapse of the lung T in parts or as a whole. This occurs in the premature infants.

Atopy (AY-top-ee) AKA Atopic syndrome: *Gk atopis = out of place* group of diseases characterized by the tendency to have a severe hypersensitive reaction to common materials in the RT, GIT &/or skin *adj. atopic = allergic* as in allergic rhinitis (hay fever) = olfactory & sinusoid mucosa IF, allergic asthma = IF of the airways & atopic dermatitis (eczema) = skin IF.

Atresia (A-treez-ee-uh): *Gk. a = negative, & tresis = a hole,* an absence or closure of a body orifice or tubular organ

atreto (a-TREE-toh)- closed, imperforate

Atrium (AY-tree-um): *Lt. = entrance hall,* adj.- atrial referring to any chambers which lie before a major chamber as in the heart *pl. - atria.*

Attrition: tooth wear & tear

Atrophy (a-TROH-fee): *Gk. a = negative, & trophe = food* wasting away deterioration of a T or organ from lack of use or food

Atypical (AY-tip-i-kal): not usual – often used to describe possible cancerous cells or T

Augmented breath: a sigh, a deep breath, having an inspirational duration >1.5s *see also MT breathing patterns*

auto- (OR-toh) self, spontaneous

Autolysis (OR-tol-e-sis): *Gk auto = self , lysis = dissolving* - hence the process of self destruction of a cell or T see **the A to Z of Major organs** for more details

aux- (ORKS) help, growth, increase

Axilla AKA Armpit AKA Underarm: *Lt. axilla = armpit* pertaining to the triangular region at the top of the UL & the upper thoracic wall – *the underarm*

Axial: refers to the head & trunk (vertebrae, ribs & sternum) of the body.

Axis (AX-is): *Lt. axis = the central line of a body or part thereof, especially the imaginary line around which rotation takes place* refers to the head & trunk (Vertebrae, Ribs & Sternum) of the body. *adj. axial (AX-see-al) pl axes*

B

bar- pressure

Baroreceptor: a sense organ responsive to stretch of the large BVs signaling BP changes

bary- low, heavy, deep difficult

Base a substance combined with protons to neutralize acids

Basement membrane (BM) a thin layer of EC material (A) containing interlocking fibrous material (B) that underlies every epithelial cell, facilitating epithelial cell movement & nutrition

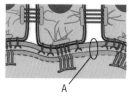
A

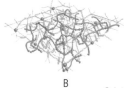
B

© A. L. Neill

basi- foundation, base

baso- base c.f. acid / base & in the bottom – the basal layer

Basophil (BAY-so-fil): *base loving - a type of WBC that is characterized by* large cytoplasmic granules that stain blue with basic dyes. *see MT*

Benign (BEE-nïn): *Fr benignus = kind* hence not harmful or dangerous, (≠ **Malignant**) indicating a mild disease or a mild non-malignant cancer

bi- twice, two, double

Bifid: *adj. Lt. bis = double, & findo = to split.*

Bifurcate: *Lt. bis = double, & furco = fork*, hence to divide into two.

Bilateral: *Lt. bi = two, lateral = side*, hence, pertaining to two (both) sides.

bin- twice , two, double

bio- (bï-oh) life

Biogenesis: the development or formation of ...e.g. biogenesis of an organelle may result from the fusion of several components ± their further modification

Biopsy (BĬ-op-see): a piece of T removed for microscopic examination – usually from a live person *see also the A to Z of Hair, Nails & Skin for more details*

blast- undifferentiated immature

Blocked nose: ↓ AF through the nose, if completely blocked – there is no AF. Both nostrils will not allow air through. If one nostril is allowing minimal air then technically the nose is congested & not blocked, although often it is referred to as "blocked" Causes include: swollen mucosa ± ↑ mucous secretions, enlarged inferior turbinates, deviated septum. *see also Nare, Nasal Congestion, Nose, Nostril*

Blood Gas Barrier (BGB): the structures separating the air in the alveoli from the site of GE – needs to be as thin as possible to allow for effective diffusion *see also MT alveoli*

Bogey (BOH-gee) slang term for Dried nasal mucosa: note ↑ AF or ↓ mucous secretions causes the superficial layer of the secretion to become harder/crusty, so that when removed it becomes semi-solid. This drying hinders the moisturizing & warming of the air through the nose & may lead to ↑ coughing. Although it is considered impolite to eat "bogeys" , there is an argument that by doing so the immune system – in particular tonsils, is exposed to normal air-bourne bacteria & functions better other slang terms include bugey, bugger

Bohr shift: the shift in the oxyHb dissoc. curve caused by a change in the pH - mainly due to the ↑ $[CO_2]$ which favours the offloading of the O_2 in the Ts & the uploading of O_2 in the lungs *see also Haldane effect*

brachy- (brak-EE) short

Branchia (BRANK-ee-uh): *Gk. = gills, adj.- branchial.*

Breathing Apparatus: Fish have gills as their breathing apparatus - O_2 is exchanged as fluid moves over the gill's surface pumped passed with fish swimming. As animals left the water, the breathing apparatus changed to reflect this, as demonstrated in the following summary of the development & variations of various breathing apparatus.

    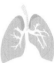

| Fish - Gills water coursing over the membranes | Amphibians - relying upon skin & lungs w/o alveolar | Reptiles - allowing for positive ventilation from rib & abdominal movement | Birds - have lungs & airsacs for GE | Mammalian - lungs with alveoli & increased SA and negative inspiration |

brevi- short

Bronchi (BRON-kee): airways b/n the trachea & alveoli - part of the dead air space *adj. bronchial; sing. bronchus*

Bronchial (BRON-kee-al) tree: reference to the appearance of the conductive airway pathways which look like the branching of a tree.

Bronchiectasis (BRON-kee-ek-tas-is): permanent dilatation (d) of the bronchi 2° to chronic In. The widened airways weaken & become filled with mucoid fluid &/or infective material (f) leaving the lung chronically inflamed. It is the end stage of many pulmonary diseases including cystic fibrosis & emphysema.

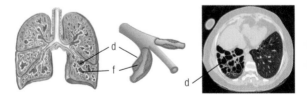

The process becomes a vicous circle of pathology

The process becomes one of an increasing positive feedback pathological process.

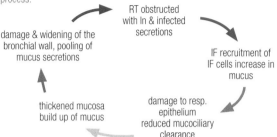

RT obstructed with In & infected secretions

IF recruitment of IF cells increase in mucus

damage to resp. epithelium reduced mucociliary clearance

thickened mucosa build up of mucus

damage & widening of the bronchial wall, pooling of mucus secretions

Bronchiolus: one of the numerous subdivisions of the intrapulmonary 2° bronchi in which the diameter is reduced to <1mm *see also MT*

Bronchitis (bron-KĬ-tis): IF of the upper airways resulting in a persistent cough, which if it is longer than 3 mnths is called chronic bronchitis

Bronchoconstriction: narrowing of the bronchi & bronchioles caused by contraction of the bronchial smooth muscle. This occurs in asthma & allergic reactions, *see MT.*

Bruxism: *Lt brukhein = gnashing of teeth* grinding of one's teeth, generally occurs unconsciously during sleep.

Bronchopneumonia: IF of the lungs producing patchy widespread consolidation

Buccal (BUK-al): pertaining to the cheek

Buffer: a system which maintains the AB balance in the body usually by absorbing & releasing the H^+ ion & the formation of the bicarbonate ion - HCO_3^-

Burp AKA Belch AKA Eructation: a NRAM - air escaping from the upper GIT, accompanied often by a sound & odour. It does not involve the RT, although because of the acid content, this may lead to *a dry hacking cough*, due to laryngeal irritation. Particularly prevalent in babies as the oesophageal sphincter is not fully formed.

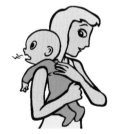

C

cac- (KAK) bad, diseased, deformed, ill

Cancer (KAN-ser): Lt crab - describing originally the crab-like invasion of cancer cells spreading out into normal T – malignant neoplasms

Cannula AS Canula (KAN-yew-lar): Lt cannula = little roof / a tube hence a tube which is inserted into the body, as in the insertion of a cannula into the larynx to keep the airway open

Capillary (kap-IL-lar-ee): Lt. capillaris = hair-like, hence a very thin BV that interconnects arterioles with venules. The capillary wall is a single cell layer in thickness, & is the only site of nutrient diffusion b/n the BS & body cells, & of GE in the lungs.

Capsule (KAPS-yew-l): Lt. capsa = box, hence an enclosing membrane

Carbminohaemoglobin (carbHb): the normal complex of Hb carrying CO_2 see **the A to Z of Blood** for more details

Carcinogen (KAR-sin-oh-jen): material which leads to cancer formation

Carcinoid: description of a tumour or agentaffin cells in various organs, slow growing & covered in mucosa

Carcinoma (KAR-sin-oh-mah): a malignant growth originating from epithelial cells

Carcinoma – in situ pre-invasive cancer still lying in the confines of normal T not having broken through the BM but with neoplastic changes

Carina (KAR-een-uh): the end of the trachea & point origin of the 2 1° bronchi. It is the site of the coughing reflex. see also MT

Carotid body: peripheral chemoreceptors at the bifurcation of the common carotid a

Cartilage (KAR-til-lej): Lt. = gristle; adj.- cartilaginous a type of CT characterized by the presence of a matrix containing a dense distribution of proteins & a thickened ground substance, (hyaline cartilage A) with many fibres - e.g. collagen (fibrocartilage B) or elastic fibres (elastic cartilage C) .

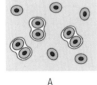
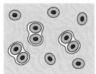
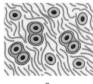

| A | B | C |

Catarrh (KAT-arh) AKA "Common Cold": Lt = catarrhus, kata down flow, is an excessive build-up of thick phlegm or mucus in an airway or cavity of the body, generally the sinuses, but also in the throat, ears or chest. It is associated with nasal congestion, sneezing, mild fever & red, weepy eyes. adj catarrhal

© A. L. Neill

Cava: *Lt. cavum = cave, hollow adj cavernous containing caverns or cave-like spaces.*

Cavity (KAV-it-ee): *Lt. cavitas = a hollow* hence an open area or sinus enclosed by a bone or boney cage c.f. the rib cage enclosing the thoracic cavity.

Cell (SELL): the basic living unit of multi-cellular organisms.

Cell body: the portion of a cell containing the nucleus & much of the cytoplasm. (AKA the soma).

Cell membrane (CM) AKA plasma membrane: the bilipid layer containing a variable number of proteins & sugars, which separates the IC from the EC environment & defines volume of a cell

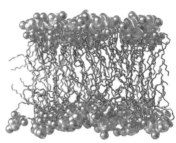

cen- general, common - new recent

centi- hundredth part, hundred

Central Chemoreceptors: chemosensitive regions of the medulla whose activity promotes breathing

cephal- head

Cephalic (KEF–al-ik): *Gk. kephale = head* pertaining to the head

cer- (ser) wax

cheil- lip (cheel-)

chemo- (keem-oh) relating to chemistry, chemically induced

Chemotaxis (KEEM-oh-tax-is): cellular phenomenon of moving towards or away from specific areas due to the chemical present

chiro- (kyro-) hand

Chloride shift: the movement of chloride ions into or out of RBCs to compensate for the movement of bicarbonate ions & so maintain electrical neutrality & AB.

chondra- (kondra-) cartilage *Gk. chondros = cartilage*

Chorda: *Lt. = cord.*

chron- (kron-) time

Chronic (KRON-ik): long standing (≠ **Acute**), generally used in disease states

Chronic Obstructive Airways Disease (COAD): a collective term for IF airway diseases (e.g. emphysema, chronic bronchitis, bronchopneumonia etc). This term is synonymous with COLD, COPD.

Cilium (sil-ee-um): *Lt cilia = eyelashes* hence hair-like process(A) associated with cells; a modification of the CM with specific internal fibrillar cytoskeletal structures which allows it independent movement as opposed to a mv(B), which does not. Ciliary movement generates a flow of fluid (usually mucus) in the EC environment. *adj. ciliary, ciliated pl. cilia*

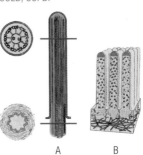

A   B

cine- (sin-ee) movement

Circadian Rhythm: the day/night cycle determined by the pineal gland through its secretion of melatonin. Sleep patterns are in part determined by the levels of melatonin. *see also Melatonin*

circum- (SER-kum) around , surrounding

cis- (sis) on this side

Clara cells: "clear & famous" cells found at the beginning of the terminal bronchioles, which produce surfactant similar to Type II cells of the alveoli. Clara cells "peg out" when they release their secretions often dying in the process - holocrine secretion *see also surfactant MT cells of respiration*

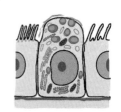

"Clearing the throat" *see Throat*

cleist- (klïst-) closed

clist- closed

Closing Volume: as the Lung Volume (LV) is reduced towards the Residual Volume (RV), there is a point when the airways start to close. Closing Vol = Closing Capacity - RV

co- (koh) with together

coen- general, common

col- with, together

Cold AKA Common Cold AKA Nasopharyngitis AKA Rhinopharyngitis AKA Coryza: an acute but mild self-limiting viral infection(s) of the URT, primarily affecting the nose & throat. SS mainly result from the body's reaction to the infectious agents include: low fever, coughing, congested/ runny nose, headache, sneezing & sore throat. Duration is b/n 3-10 days or if severe up to 21 days. The cough may persist for longer. The rhinoviruses are the commonest causes, although >200 viruses have been implicated, often occurring together i.e. the cold may result from multiple viral Ins & lead onto a bacterial In.

coelom- (SEE-lohm) body cavity

Collagen (KOL-a-jen): a protein that is an abundant component of CT.

Collateral: *adj. Lt. con = together & latus = side*, hence, alongside.

Columna: *Lt. = column, or pillar.*

com- together, with

Coma (KOH-mah): *Gk koma = sleep* hence refers to a depressed state of consciousness & ability to respond to stimuli. The breathing patterns change with varied conscious states - *see MT breathing patterns*

Compliance: the ease of stretching the lungs or the chest wall. Reduced in fluid filled walls - which occurs with RV failure / pulmonary oedema (≠ **Elastance**).

con- together with

Concha (KONG-ku) AKA Turbinate: a shell shaped bone as in the ear or nose *pl. conchae adj. chonchoid.*

Conductance: the ease with which the gas or liquid can be made to flow through a tube (≠ **Resistance**).

Conducting airways: the airways which conduct the gas to the site of GE. These passages make up most of the ADS, & are proximal to the respiratory bronchioles.

Congenital (KON-jen-it-al): present from birth

Connective tissue (CT) (kon-EK-tiv Tish-ew): one of the 4 basic types of T in the body. It is characterized by an abundance of EC material with relatively few cells, & functions in the support & binding of body structures.

Consolidation: term used to describe when the normally air filled alveoli in the lung become solid with cells &/or exudate etc - present in pneumonias V/Q<1 approaching zero in severe cases.

Constrictor: to squeeze - generally referring to a circular muscle's action where it ↓ the size of an opening often to direct movement of the contents in a single direction (as in Pharynx, with swallowing) *see also Sphincter*

Continuous Airways Positive Pressure (CPAP): a method of non invasive ventilation whereby air is blown into the airways for the whole respiratory cycle. It is generally delivered via a mask over the mouth &/or nose for sufferers of OSA, pushing open the soft palate.

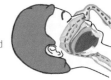

contra- opposite against

Contralateral: *Lt. contra = against, latus = side*, the opposite side (≠ **Ipsilateral**)

cor- heart

Cor pulmonare: RV enlargement due to pulmonary hypertension *see also Pulmonary Hypertension*

Cornu: a horn (as in the Hyoid)

Corona (kor-ROH-nuh): *Lt. coron = crown, hence, encircling like a crown*: a crown. *adj. coronary, coronoid or coronal*; hence a coronal plane is parallel to the main arch of a crown which passes from ear to ear (*c.f. coronal suture*). It extends vertically to divide the body into ant. & post. portions, AKA the frontal plane

corp- (kor) body

Corpus: *Lt. = body, pl.- corpora*. pertaining to the body or the main part of the organ

Corpuscle (KOR-puhs-el): *Lt. = a little body* hence used to describe a small body contained w/n a sac, as in red corpuscle (RBC) small package of Hb

Coryza (KOR-ĭ-zuh) AKA Cold AKA Rhinitis

Cortex (KOR-tehks): *Lt. = bark, adj. cortical* the outer portion of an organ. (≠ **Medulla**)

cost- (kost) rib *Lt. = rib. adj. costal*

Cough (KOF): non-respiratory air movement due to forced expiration against a closed glottis *see MT*

Countercurrent: two streams flowing in an opposite directions to maximize the exchange of chemicals or heat

Cribriform / Ethmoid: a sieve or bone with small sieve-like holes.

Cricoid: a ring wrt pulmonary system the uppermost ring of the trachea – & the only complete tracheal ring. It is associated with the thyroid & arytenoid cartilages and larynx *see also arytenoid cartilages, larynx.*

-crine (krïn) to secrete

crur-(kroo-r) leg *Lt. = leg, sing crus pl - crura.*

crypt- hidden, covered occult

Cutis - (KEW-tis): *Lt. cutis = the skin adj cutaneous (kew-TAY-nee-us)*

Cyanosis (SĬ-an–oh-sis): *Gk kyanos –blue material*, hence blueness mauveness of the skin, or elsewhere due to the amounts of de-oxygenated Hb

cyst- (sist-) sac, bladder

Cyst (sist-): *Gk. kystis = bladder, adj. cystic*. referring to fluid enclosed w/n epidermal layers c.f. cystic fibrosis

Cystic Fibrosis (CF): an autosomal recessive condition caused by a defect(td) in the cystic fibrosis transmembrane transporter(t) of the Chloride ion(c) resulting in the abnormally viscous lung secretions(sv), due to the fact that water(w) travels back into the absorptive cells(a) rather than remaining in the airways & diluting the coating mucous(m). This causes the lungs to be prone to Ins & bronchiectasis, even though other ion transporters(o) are not affected.

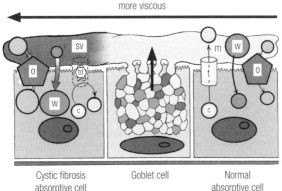

more viscous

| Cystic fibrosis absorptive cell | Goblet cell | Normal absorptive cell |

In the bronchioles this presents as dilated damaged walls(B - 5d) with cilia(2) damaged or missing (2d) full of mucus(1). The number of mucous glands(3) is unchanged but the secretions do not move on, which damages the lining epitheium(4).

Cystic fibrosis also affects the pancreas sectretions & production of semen.
see also Bronchiectasis

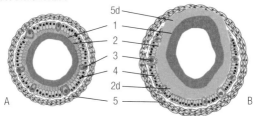

5d
1
2
3
4
2d
5

A   B

cyto-/-cyte (sĭt-OH-) cell mature cell type

Cytoplasm (SĪ-to-plazm): the material of a cell located w/n the CM & outside the NM containing the cellular organelles.

Cytosol (SĪ-toh-sol) the thickened fluid of the cytoplasm. It lies outside the cellular organelle membranes.

Cytoskeleton (sī-toh-SKEL-eh-ton): the complex supportive network of microtubules & microfilaments in the cytoplasm. *For more details see **the A to Z of Major organs***

D

de- remove, undoing, reversal, depriving, freeing from

Dead Space (DS): areas in the RT which do not have any GE - ↑ in many disease states & in CCF *see also Consolidation*

dec- (des) ten, tenth

Deglutition: *Lt. deglutire = to swallow*, hence the act of swallowing.

Degranulation: the process of shedding granules from the cell cytoplasm into the exterior (c.f. degranulation of mast cells in an allergic reaction)

dem- people, population

demi- (dem-ee) half

Dendrite AKA Dendron: *Gk. = a tree*, hence like the branches of a tree.

dendro- branching, treelike

Dens: a tooth, denticulate having tooth-like projections *adj dental, dentate, dentine denticulate*

Depress: *Lt. de = prefix implying descent & pressum = pressed*, hence to press down

Depression: downward movement or a concavity on a surface.

Dermatome *Gk. derma = skin, tome = a cutting or division*, a segment of skin supplied by a single SN *see also Myotome.*

derm(o)- skin

Dermatitis (derm-u-TĬ-tis): any skin IF

di two, twice, double, reversal , separation, apart from

dia- through across, between , apart , complete

Diaphragm: *Gk. dia = across, & phragma = wall*, hence, a partition. Generally this refers to the dome-shaped muscular sheet which separates the thorax from the abdomen, *adj. diaphragmatic*

Diffuse parenchymal lung disease AKA Interstitial lung disease: diseases where the interstitium is thickened generally by fibrosis, ↓ GE. These diseases maybe idiopathic but are often associated with IF diseases & IF caused by breathing in FBs such as asbestos, silicon & carbon particles

Diffusing Capacity: the ability of the lung to allow gas to diffuse from the air to the B & vv

Diffusion: the process whereby a substance is transported along a concentration gradient by a random movement of molecules

diplo- double, twin

dis- apart from, two, twice, double , reversal, separation, difficult, wrong

Discharge: the term used to imply the oozing of a mucoid liquid e.g. nose, throat

Discus (DIS-kus): *Lt. = disc. adj. discoid*

Disease (DIZ-eez): *Eng. dis- ease = lack of comfort,* anything limiting health & comfort of the organism

Distal (DIS-tahl): *Lt. di = apart & stans = standing,* away from the middle of the body or the axis or core of the body ($\neq$ proximal)

Dorsum (DOR-sal): *Lt. dorsum = back adj = dorsal* a directional term indicating toward the back side, or posterior

Drive to breathe: physiological changes which increase ventilation c.f. $\downarrow$ O_2 &/or $\uparrow$ CO_2
In most people the drive to breathe depends upon the B[CO_2], rather than the O_2 levels. Oxygen drive occurs in long standing patients with COAD as the B[CO_2] is constantly elevated, and o no longer a reliable parameter.

duo- (DEW-oh) two

dy- two

Dynamic Airway Collapse: collapse of the airways provoked by $\uparrow$ flow c.f. coughing $\uparrow$ flow & collapse

dys- (dis) difficult, painful, abnormal

Dysplasia: changes in the morphology of growing cells / Ts

Dyspnoea: the sensation of breathlessness - irregular breathing

Dystrophy (DIS-troh-fee): irregular abnormal growth

E

e- outside external out protrude over away less

ec- outside out to protrude over away less / house

Ectasia (EK-tay-zee-yuh): dilatation or distention of a tubular structure. Maybe physiological & under H influence e.g. duct ectasia of the breast, a dilated milk duct, or pathological c.f. bronchi / bronchiole ectasia.

ecto- outer out of place

-ectomy to cut out , excise surgically

Ectoderm (EHK-toh-derm): *Gk. ektos = outside & derm = skin* the outermost layer of the 3 primary germ layers in the developing embryo. It gives rise to the NS & to the epidermis & its derivatives

Edema (eh –DEE-mah) AS Oedema

Edentulous: w/o teeth

Edge: border or margin of a surface.

ef- outside out to protrude over away less

Efferent: *adj. Lt. ex = out, & ferens = carrying*, hence, conducting from. Efferent Ns move away from the brain - & are motor Ns ≠ **Afferent**

Elastance ≠ Compliance

Elastic recoil: the tendency of the lungs to resist stretching, due to their elasticity

Elasticity (ee-laz-STIS ih-tee): the physiological property of T to return to its original shape after distortion

Elastin: major EC fibre which has large recoil properties - made up of fibrillin(1) filaments & elastin matrix(2). These assemble EC after smaller IC components are extruded.

Later X-links form in the EC, adding to its elastic properties.

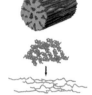

Emphysema (EMPF-uh-seem-uh): defined as the anatomical destruction of the alveolar septa resulting in permanent enlargement of the air spaces distal to the terminal bronchioles. Part of the spectrum of COAD. The result is permanently hyperinflated lungs - with reduced elastic recoil - so that expiration is difficult to complete.

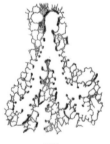
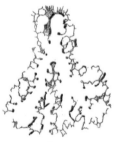

NAD   emphysema

em- within, inside, into in on

Embolus (EM-bohl-us): *Gk embolos = plug, wedge or blocking matter* hence a mass which travels in the BS & suddenly blocks an artery i.e. plugs it up, frequently resulting from a dislodged thrombus. If this arises from the LL then it may lodge in the pulmonary arteries causing sudden SOB ± death - pulmonary embolus *adj emboliformis see also Thrombosis*

emet- vomiting

-emia AS –aemia pertaining to blood, generally RBCs

en- within, inside, in, on

endo- within, inside, into, on

Endocytosis (ehn'-do-sih-TO-sihs): the active process of bulk transport of material into a cell. It includes phagocytosis & pinocytosis.

Endoderm (en-DOH-derm): *Gk. endo = within, & derm = skin* one of the 3 primary germ layers in an embryo, it begins as the inner layer, later forms the organs of the DT & the RT.

Endoplasmic reticulum (ER) (en-doh-PLAZ-mik reh-TIK-yew-lum): a cytoplasmic organelle that consists of a series of tubules with a hollow center. It functions in the transport of cellular products (smooth ER), & as a site for protein synthesis (if ribosomes are attached, called rough ER)

Endothelium (en-doh-THEE-lee-um): *Gk. endo = within, & thele = the nipple* a layer of simple squamous epithelium lining the inside of BVs & the heart chambers.

Endotoxins AKA Lipopolysacchardies (LPS) AKA Lipoglycans: *Gk. endo = within, & toxia = poison*, are large molecules consisting of a lipid(1) & a polysaccharide(2) composed of O-Ag(2O), an outer core(2o) & inner core(2i). They are found in the CM of Gram-negative bacteria, (e.g. *Bordetella Pertussis*) & elicit a strong IR, AKA septic shock due mainly to the lipid component. ↑ adj endotoxic shock

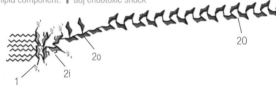

ent-   within, inner

Eosinophil (ee-oh-SIN-oh-fil): a type of granulated WBC characterized by a cytoplasm which absorbs the eosin stain. *see MT*

ep-   upon, in addition to, beside among, on the outside, over

epi-   upon, in addition to, beside, among, on the outside, over

Epidural: *adj.Gk. epi = upon, Lt. dura = tough*, hence, external to the dura mater (DM).

Epiglottis: an unpaired leaf like plate of fibro elastic cartilage Vallecula situated behind the root of the tongue (lingual surface - 1) & Hyoid & in front of the laryngeal inlet (laryngeal surface - 2) attached to the thyroid cartilage by the petiolus (cartilaginous stem - 3)

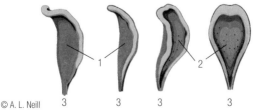

Epistaxis: nosebleed, generally from the septum in the Little's area an intersection of the 3 main BVs supplying the nose

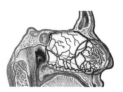

equi- equal

Equal Pressure point: during forced expiration that point of the airways where the intraluminal P = the external lung P, & collapse is likely to occur

-ergy action

erythr- red

Erythema (eh-REE-thee-muh): *Gk.: flushing on the skin – redness*

Erythrocyte AKA red blood cell (RBC): anucleate biconcave cell, the commonest in circulating B which acts as a carrier of O_2 & CO_2 through its Hb.

Ethmoidectomy: removal of the partitions b/n the ethmoid sinuses (A) creating larger sinus cavities (B) to treat/cure chronic sinusitis caused by repeated sinus Ins & obstructions, which are often associated with nasal polyps.

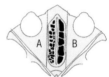

Ethmoids AKA ethmoid sinuses *(slang)* air spaces in the Ethmoid bone b/n the eyeballs, extending to the bridge of the nose, & drains into the nasal cavity. If fluid is trapped in this area, it may cause chronic infections & sinusitis & may require an ethmoidectomy.

eu- good normal well easily

eury- broad wide

Eversion: *Lt. e = out, and versum = turned*, hence turned outwards.

ex- to protrude outside out over away less

Excretion (ek-SKREE-shun): the processes by which metabolic waste materials are removed from cells, Ts or entire bodies.

exo- outside outer layer out of

Expiratory Flow Limitation: the point where in expiration – it is not possible to force more air out as the lung Ts have collapsed this ↑ with age & disease meaning there is less working volume for GE in the lung

External: *adj. Lt. externus = outward*, hence, further from the inside.

External Auditory Meatus (EAM): ear hole

extra- outside of out over beyond, in addition to,

Extracellular environment (EKS-trah-CEL-yew-lar en-VĬ-ROH-ment): the body space outside the CM.

Extracellular fluid (ECF): the fluid outside the CM, including interstitial fluid & B plasma.

F

Facet (FASS-et): a face, a small bony surface (occlusal facet on the chewing surfaces of the teeth) seen in planar joints.

faci- (fasi)   to do with the face

fasci- (fashi-)   band, connection

Fascia (FASH-ee-ah): *Lt. = band or bandage* a sheet or band of dense CT that structurally supports organs & Ts. Deep fascia surrounds muscle, & superficial fascia separates the skin & muscle layers. *adj. fascial*

Fauces (FOR-seez): jaws or throat

febri-   fever

fila-   threadlike thread

Filament *see also microfilament*: a single thread or strand which may be thick or thin but is not made up of obvious multiple units as may be the case in a fibre

Fibre AS fiber *see also Filament*: a rope or long strand of material - may have multiple subfibres or filaments in its makeup or appear as a single unit in biology there are 4 main types - the collagens; the elastins, the fibrillins & the fibronectins, but the most important by far is the collagen group *adj. fibrillar*

Fissure (FISH-er): a narrow slit or gap from cleft.

Flexure (FLEX-shew-er): *Lt. flexura = a bending.*

Forced Vital Capacity (FVC): the largest breath possible

Forced Expiratory Volume in 1 sec (FEV$_1$): the volume of air a subject can blow from maximum inspiration in 1 second. This is used to assess AR.

fore-   front or before

Fossa (FOS-ah): *Lt. = a ditch or trench* hence a depression or concavity on bones or organs formed by several bones

Fovea: *Lt. = a pit* (usually smaller than a fossa).

fract-   break

Free radicals: unbound charged ions or molecules - highly reactive *see also Radicals*

Frenulum: *Lt. = bridle or curb* (diminutive of frenum), it is a CT band which anchors one moving layer to another fixed T e.g. in the mouth it anchors the tongue.

Functional Residual Capacity (FRC): the volume of air remaining in the lungs when forced expiration is complete

G

Gag Reflex AKA Pharyngeal reflex AKA Laryngeal spasm: is a contraction of the back of the throat triggered by an object touching the roof of your mouth, the back of your tongue, the area around your tonsils, or the back of your throat

Gargle: wash one's mouth & throat with a liquid that is kept in motion by breathing air through it from the lungs with a gurgling sound. This is an example of NRAM

Gasp (GARSP): rapid intake of breath due to something unexpected, another NRAM

Generation: wrt the pulmonary system – the level of branching of the respiratory tree, beginning with the Trachea as generation 0 & the initial branching of the primary bronchi as generation 1/ lobar bronchi as 2 & 3, segmental bronchi as 4…alveolar sacs are then generation 23 *see MT*

Gingiva (JIN-jiv-uh): *Lt. gingiva = gums* gum

Gland: *Lt. glans = an acorn, adj. glandular* a specialization of epithelial T to secrete substances. It may consist of a single cell or a multi-cellular arrangement.

Glottis: *Gk. glotta = tongue* the space b/n the vocal cords & structures involved in the production of the voice; inner part of the larynx. The surrounding structures are the Rima Glottides, the space is the Glottis – note the Epiglottis sits above the glottis acting as a roof when the Hyoid is raised in swallowing, otherwise it sits upright exposing the tracheal lumen pl. glottedis / glottisses

Glycan (GLĪ-kan): a sugar

H

Haeme AS Heme blood, This is the complex which is housed in a large globular protein to form Hb

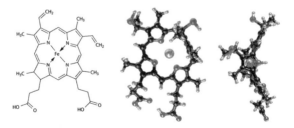

Haematocrit (hee-MAT-o-krit): the percentage of RBCs in a sample of B, which is determined by centrifuging the sample & measuring the RBC volume relative to other B components.

Haematopoiesis (heem-ah-to-poy-EE-sihs): the production of B cells in the red bone marrow. **(also = haemopoiesis. AS hematopoiesis)**

Haemoglobin (Hb) (HEE-mo-glo-bihn): a complex protein inside the RBCs involved in the transport of O_2 & CO_2. It is present in the B in many forms:.
cyanohaemoglobin,
deoxyhaemoglobin deoxyHb, / oxyhaemoglobin – oxyHb, &
methaemoglobin - metHb.
Each molecule has 4 active centres, each housing the haeme complex, which is bound & so positioned that its iron ion (Fe) centre is exposed. Other molecules bind to these centres - as in O2 with oxy-Hb. *For more details see the A to Z of Blood*

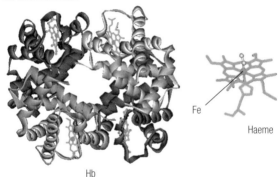

Fe

Haeme

Hb

Haemoptysis: coughing up B

Haemorrhage (Hg) (HEM-or-rij): *Gk haeme = blood , rhegnymi = to burst forth,* loss of B outside the CVS

Haldane effect: deoxygenated B has a higher capacity to carry CO_2 than oxygenated B. This allows more venous B to carry away CO_2 from the Ts. *see also Bohr Effect*

Halitosis AKA Bad breath AKA Fetor Oris

Hay fever AKA Allergic rhinitis

Heat of Evaporation: the amount of heat needed to cause 1g of a liquid to evaporate – with water this is high & hence evaporating water from the skin has a cooling effect

hemi-   half

Henderson- Hasselbalch equation: the equation which relates B pH to the B[CO_2] & B[HCO_3]. It is a poor estimation of pH in either strong acids or bases, because it relies upon a number of assumptions. The most significant is that the concentration of the acid & its conjugate base at equilibrium & will remain the same as the formal concentration.
In the Henderson–Hasselbalch equation the B[pH] is related to the constituents of the bicarbonate buffering system

Hiccup AS Hiccough AKA Singultus AKA Synchronous diaphragmatic flutter: an involuntary spasm (myoclonic jerk) of the diaphragm followed by a sudden closure of the glottis (vocal chords) causing the "Hik" & interrupting the normal breathing cycle, & releasing air from the stomach. Hiccups involve the repetition of stimulation of a reflex arc involving the pharyngeal branch of the Glossopharyngeal N ➜ Phrenic N (NRs C345), & occur predominantly in infants or after neurological damage, as single or multiple events - bouts of hiccups. *see also MT non respiratory air movements*

Hilum (HĪ-lum): the small space, gap or notch in an organ where vessels & other structures may enter & leave - wrt pulmonary system the hilum of the lung AKA the root of the lung. It is the site of entrance of all the BVs NS lymphatics & bronchi of the lungs.

holo-   entire

Holocrine: secretions which involve the death of the cell with substance liberation *see also Clara cells*

homo-   same

homeo (HOHM-ee-oh)   same common like

horm-   to urge, to stimulate

Hyaline cartilage (HĪ-al-ĭn): a type of CT that contains chondrocytes embedded w/n lacunae, both of which are surrounded by a dense, semi translucent matrix of collagen fibers & glycosaminoglycans.

hydr- (hĭdr)   water

hygr-water

Hyoid: *adj. Gk. hyoeides =* U-shaped. U-shaped bone - with a body(1) with small horns (cornu)(2) & large horns(3). It is the only bone which does not articulate, with any other in the body. It is raised in swallowing to push the epiglottis forward and shut off the trachea, directing food into the oesophagus.

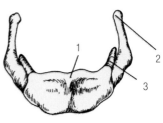

hyper - (hĭ-per)   excessive ≠ hypo

Hypercapnia: an elevated B[CO_2] ≠ **Hypocapnia**

Hyperplasia (HĬ-per-PLAY-zee-ar): ↑ production & growth of cells beyond normal limits.

Hypersomnolence: too much sleep to the extent it is interfering with daily activities

Hypertonic (HĬ-per-TON-ik): the state of a solution having a greater concentration of dissolved particles than the solution it is compared to (≠ **Hypotonic**).

Hypertrophy (hï-PER-troh-fee): the abnormal enlargement or growth of a cell, T, or organ.

hypo- deficient below under ≠ hyper

Hypodermis (hï-po-DERM-is): the area of the body b/n the dermis of the skin & skeletal muscle

Hypoventilation: insufficient ventilation of the alveoli to maintain normal B[CO_2] & B[O_2] levels

Hypoxaemia: ↓ B[O_2] – in particular arterial B

Hypoxia: inadequate levels of O_2 in the cells / Ts

Hypoxic vasoconstriction: the constriction of pulmonary BVs in response to alveolar ↓ [O_2] levels. This prevents the over-perfusion of under-ventilated regions. In the systemic BVs ↓ [O_2] causes vasodilatation

I

iatr- (ee-at-rah) to treat

ictero- (IK-ter-oh) jaundiced

Idiopathic (ID-ee-oh-path- ik): *Gk. = idios one's self, pathos sickness* a spontaneous sickness or illness of unknown origin (= Agnogenic)

ile - pertaining to the ileum

im- in, into, on, onto, not, non

In parallel: elements or tubes which take flow or move in the same direction at the same time & are connected at both ends FLOW α 1/RESISTANCE ≠ **in series**

infero- low, lower

Inferior (ihn-FER-ee-or): *Lt. = lower down* a directional term describing a location

Inflammation (IF) (in-FLAM-ay-shon): body response to any T damage caused by exposure of arachidonic acid from ruptured CMs.

Influenza AKA 'flu: an infectious disease caused by an influenza virus. SS include: a high fever, nasal congestion, coughing, sore throat, headache, muscle aches & pains, fatigue, ± nausea which begin 2-3 days after exposure to the virus, & last for 2-3 weeks. Three types of influenza viruses affect people, called Type A, Type B, and Type C, but these viruses can evolve rapidly, so that vaccinations have to be updated regularly. *see also the Cold*

infra- (infruh) below, beneath

inter - between

Intercellular (in-ter-SEL-yoo-lar): the area b/n cells.

Intercostal (IC): the space bordered by 2 ribs - defined as space b/n rib 3 & 4 is IC space 3

Interstitial fluid (ihn-tehr-STIH-shool FLOO-id): the portion of EC fluid which fills the T spaces b/n cells.

Interstitial lung disease (ILD) AKA Diffuse parenchymal disease: a diverse group of lung diseases which involve the interstitium / parenchyma of the lung - i.e. the T extending from the alveolar epithelium to the capillary endothelium. e.g. Cystic Fibrosis *see also Cystic fibrosis*

Interstitium: material including cells, b/n 2 different parenchyma

Intervertebral disk: a cartilaginous joint consisting of a pad of fibrocartilage located b/n two adjacent vertebrae.

Intima: *Lt. = innermost.*

intra- (in-truh) *Lt. = within* **within**

Intrapleural: w/n the 2 pleural layers or pleural cavity

Introitus: *Lt. intro = within, & ire = to go,* i.e. an orifice or point of entry to a cavity or space e.g. tracheal introitus.

Inversion: *Lt. = in, & vertere = to turn,* hence to turn inward, inside out, upside down.

Ions (Ī-ons): charged atoms *see also Free Radicals, Radicals*

- -ve charge - anions - generally non-metal e.g. HCO_3-, Cl-,

+ve charge - cations generally metal e.g. Ca^{2+}, $Fe^{3+/2+}$, Na^+ & also H^+

ipsi- same

Ipsilateral: *Lt. ipsi = self, the same, & latus = side,* hence on the same side.

Irritant receptor AKA rapidly adapting receptor AKA deflation receptor: free N endings of small myelinated afferent Ns found in the airway walls. They provoke coughing, rapid shallow breathing & augmented breaths depending on their site

isch- suppression, blocking

Ischaemia (is-KEEM-ee-ya): result of sudden decrease in the BS to cells or Ts

Isotonic solution: a solution that contains an equal amount of solutes relative to another, hence there is no diffusion gradient or directional movement of ions or molecules.

Isthmus: *Gk. = isthmos - a narrow passage.* as in the thyroid gland the strip of T b/n the 2 main lobes

K

-kine- move

-kines stimulation of, activation for, division or growth of cells

Kyphosis (KĬ-foh-sis) AKA
Humpback: *Gk. kyphos = bent or bowed forward.* excessive outward curvature of the thoracic spine, causing hunching of the back, which may have an impact on respiration, by restricting the rib movement, partic if medically significant > 50°. This condition may be congenital but it also increases with age & bad posture, & is caused by anterior erosion of the bodies of the vertebrae. It is commonly seen in osteoporosis. *see also Scoliosis*

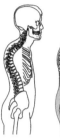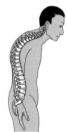

L

labi- lip

Labrum: *Lt. = rim.*

Lacrima (LAK-rim-u): related to tears & tear drops. adj. lacrimal

lacri- (LAK-ree): *Lt. lacrima = a tear (drop): adj. lacrimal*

lal- talking

Lamina (lah-MIN-uh): *Lt. lamina = plate*, hence a plate as in the lamina of the vertebra a plate of bone connecting the vertical & transverse spines or a CT membrane *adj. laminar pl. laminae* **(lah-MIN-ee)**

Laminar flow: describes the flow in a vessel which moves parallel to the BV walls w/o turbulence i.e. blood in BVs or air in airways, with smooth walls

Laplace relationship: the relationship b/n P w/n a bubble to its radius (R) & the surface tension (St) of the liquid of which it is made **P = 2St/R** hence it is harder to maintain larger bubbles that smaller ones, even with surfactant (Sp). This impacts on the alveoli, as they expand, making it more & more difficult to do so. The amount of Sp is unchanging but the surface area ↑ so even though Sp causes reduced St it is less effective in expanded inspired alveoli. *see also Surfactant*

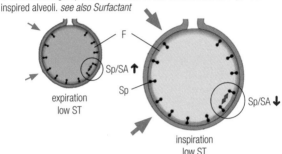

F
Sp/SA ↑
Sp

expiration
low ST

Sp/SA ↓

inspiration
low ST

Laryngitis: IF of the larynx which often results swollen VCs resulting in voice loss.

Laryngomalacia: softening of the larynx mainly the epiglottis(1) which does not stand upright, interfering with airflow in inspiration(B) & expiration(C). More prevalent in Down's syndrome & other congenital diseases. This can lead to a number of breathing difficulties - particularly in infections & sleeping.

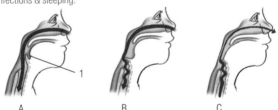

A   B   C

Larynospasm: reflex spasm of the laryngeal sphincter partic the glottic sphincter which is generally triggered by the threat of inhalation of a foreign body.

Larynx (LA-rinx) AKA Voice box: *Gk larunx = upper throat / windpipe* tubular organ extending from the root of the tongue & the Hyoid to the trachea, consisting of a cartilage framework overlaid & connected by ligs, membranes & muscles & involved in voice production *adj. laryngeal (la-rin-JEE-al)* pl = larynges, larynxes

Lata: *Lt. latus = side. adj Lateral (LAT-er-awl)* hence nearer the side a directional term describing a structure that is located further from the vertical midline of the body relative to another

Levator: to raise - generally in reference to the actions of muscles

leio- (LĬ-oh) smooth

Lesion (LEE-zshen): a destructive change in the T – such as an IF, injury or wound

leuco- white, colourless, pale

leuko- white, colourless, pale

levator- to lift up ≠ depressor

levo- left

liga- bind

Ligament (LIG-uh-ment): Lt. ligamentum = bandage a band or cord of dense CT that extends from one bone to another - tying it together to provide a joint with structural stability adj. ligamentous.

lingu- tongue see also gloss-

Lingua (ling-GEW-uh): Lt. = tongue, adj. lingual. pertaining to the tongue. c.f. the lingual frenulum connects the tongue to the floor of the mouth

Lingula: diminutive of lingua, hence, a little tongue, adj. lingular.

lio- (LĬ-oh) smooth

lip- fat

Lipopolysacchardies (LPS) AKA Endotoxins

lith- stone

Livid: Lt = lividus lead coloured – discolouration from a contusion or congested pooled B adj. livedo

Loading region: flat upper region of the oxyHb curve where O_2 can be loaded into the RBC see **the A to Z of Blood** for more information

Lobe (LOH-b): Gk. lobos = lobe, adj.- lobar. roundish projection of any structure, wrt pulmonary system: the lungs have 2 lobes on the L & 3 lobes on the R, each with their own BS & NS - functional units

Lobules (lob-YOOL): little lobe

loc- location place

Locus (LOH-kus): Lt. = a place (cf. location, locate, dislocate).

longus- long

Lumen (LOO-men) Lt. = opening the potential space w/n a tubular structure.

Lung Capacities & Volumes see MT

Lymph (LIMpf): excess fluid & proteins left behind from the capillaries as they move from the arterial to the venous side see also MT pulmonary circulation

M

macro- (MAK-roh) big

Macrophage (MAK-roh-fahrj): a large phagocytic cell originating from a monocyte *see MT.*

magna- large, great

Major (MAY-jaw): bigger of the 2 things e.g. Pectoralis major m lying over Pectoralis minor m - bigger & more supf.

mal- abnormal bad

Malar: cheek

Malignant (MAL-ig-nant): fast moving & often harmful e.g. malignant hypertension (HP) is rapidly increasing HP, with cancer it is fast growing & invading

meat- opening

Meatus (mee-AY-tus): *Lt. = passage; adj. meatal* canal, opening passage, particularly if opening onto a body surface

Mechanoreceptor: Receptors sensitive to mechanical stimulation, generally referring to Stretch receptor; wrt pulmonary system these receptors lie in: the chest wall, diaphragm, airways & respiratory mucosa. They respond to expansion of the chest wall limiting the extent of inspiration.

medi- middle intermediate

Medial (MEE-dee-al): *Lt. medius = middle adj. medial* a directional term describing a part lying nearer to the vertical midline of the body relative to another part.

Median: *Lt. medianus = in the middle.*

Mediastinum: *Lt = middle class* a medial septum b/n 2 parts of an organ or cavity wrt thorax - it is the structures contained in the middle b/n the 2 lungs & contains the great vessels, heart, LNs, Vagus & phrenic Ns, oesophagus, & trachea *see MT.*

Medulla (meh-DUL-ah): an inner, or deeper, part of an organ. e.g. the medulla of the kidneys, the medulla of the adrenal gland & the lymph node. (≠ **Cortex**)

Medulla Oblongata (MO): caudal portion of the Brainstem b/n the Pons & rostral part of the SC & contains receptors which control the breathing cycle when at rest *for more details see* **the A to Z of the Brain and Cranial Nerves**

Melatonin:
is a H secreted by the pineal gland. It maintains the body's circadian rhythm, ↑ in the dark & ↓ in the light, via the hypothalamic-pituitary axis. *for more details see **the A to Z of Endocrinology***

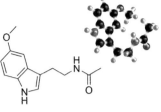

Sunlight(1) suppresses the stimulation of melatonin(3) from the pineal gland(2), causing wakefulness via the hypothalamus(4) which through the pituitary gland(5) releases ACTH causing the adrenal gland(6) to release cortisol & other stimulants(7). As the day progresses & the light wanes melatonin levels increase(8) suppressing the hypothalamic secretions causing sleepiness. Other factors also contribute to this including the feedback loop(7) &stimulants from higher centres(1o).

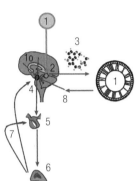

It is a strong antioxidant, which supports the immune system, & helps control the timing & release of female reproductive Hs.

Membrane (MEM-brayn): *Lt. membrana = a thin sheet; adj.- membranous* a thin sheet of tissue that lines or covers body structures. It may contain a thin layer of CT ± epithelium *see also cell membrane (CM)*

Mesial: along the dental arch in the direction of the medial plane anteriorly ≠ **Distal**

Mesoderm (MEEZ-oh-derm): *Gk. mesos = middle, & derma = skin* the middle of the three primary germ layers in a developing embryo that forms the muscles, the heart, BVs, & the CT.

Mesothelioma: cancer of the lung pleura almost always caused by asbestosis exposure

Mesothelium (mez-oh-THEE-lee-um): a simple squamous epithelium lining parts of the body's ventral cavity. *see cells of the RT*

Methaemoglobin (metHb): is a form of the oxygen-carrying metalloprotein Hb, in which the iron in the haeme group is in the Fe^{3+}(ferric) state, not the Fe^{2+}(ferrous) of normal Hb. It cannot bind O_2, unlike oxyHb. It is a chocolate brown colour & needs an enzyme - *methaemoglobin reductase (diaphorase I)* to convert it back to Hb. Only 1-2% of the Hb in the B is in this form. Any more is pathological. *see also Haemoglobin*

meta- subsequent, transformation, between, changing after

micro- small

Microvilli (mv) (mǐ-kroh-VIL-ee): microscopic extensions of the CM filled with cytoplasm that serve to increase the absorptive SA of the cell.

mid- middle

Midsagittal (MID-saj-ih-tal): a plane that extends vertically through the body, dividing it into equal R & L portions. *see also parasagittal*

Miliary: grain-like, describing small millet seed like lesions, c.f. as in miliary TB

milli- thousandth

Minimal air: the small amount of air left in the lungs, which if removed will cause alveolar collapse

Molecule: a neutral group of atoms held together by ionic or covalent bonds - however it is often also a term used for a charged polyatomic group which are technically *see also Radicals*

Monocyte (MON-oh-sǐt): a large, agranular WBC that is phagocytic. If the cell moves out from the BS into the T, it is called a macrophage, *see MT cells of Respiration.*

morph- (morf) shape

Mucociliary clearance AKA mucociliated transport AKA mucociliary escalator: the combination of mucus secretions with ciliary movement to move small particles up the RT past the epiglottis & into the DT

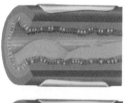

If this is suppressed, as in tobacco smoking, by the death of the cilia, the mucoid secretions thicker & drier causing ↑ AR, ↑ consolidation in the LRT leading onto bronchitis, bronchiectasis & other forms of lung consolidation.

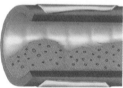

Mucophagy: the act of eating mucus from the person themselves &/or other animals

Mucopolysaccharide: a polysaccharide that contains amino sugars or monosaccharides alone or in combination with proteins.

Mucosa (MEW-koh-zuh): T immediately beneath the BM of the epithelium in the RT or DT – equivalent to the dermis in the skin

Mucous: *adj of mucus* as in mucous glands – glands which produce mucus

Mucus (MEW-kus): substance excreted by Mucous glands &/or goblet cells to lubricate food or protect mucosal surfaces as in the nasal & respiratory tracts generally clear & viscous - but it may change colours in Ins & allergic reactions, from cream through to green & yellow *adj mucous see also Phlegm*

multi- (mul-TEE-) many

Muscle Spindle: a proprioceptor which detects striated muscle length & rate of shortening. *see the A to Z of Skeletal Muscles for more details*

myc- (mïs-) fungal

myo- (mï-oh) muscle

Myotome (MĬ-oh-tome): *Gk. mys = muscle, & tome = a cutting*; a group of muscles innervated by a single SN root. *see also Dermatome & the A to Z of Peripheral Nerves for more details*

myx- (mix) mucoid

N

narco- (NARK-oh) stupor

Naris: nostrils *pl. Nares*

Naris AKA Nostril: openings of the nose for ventilation & olfaction (breathing & smelling). *pl. Nares.* There are several shapes - as infants(A) the nose is more rounded, as the cartilage is not fully formed & the fibrous T soft, hence it can be easily compressed which may have an impact on breathing in the infant - this narrows to firmer, more slotted nostrils in many adults, as the nasal septum lengthens & the fibrous T hardens(B,C) .

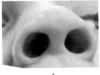

A   B   C

Nasal Congestion AKA Blocked, runny &/or stuffy noses: when there is an obstruction to the passage of air through the nose. This may be due to ↑ nasal secretions ± swelling of the conchae ± tonsillar T in particular the adenoids *see also Nose, Turbinate*

Nasal Polyps: outgrowths of the mucosal linings in the nose (A) & sinuses e.g. ethmoidal sinus polyps (B). They can be confused with the turbinates superior(s), middle(m) or inferior (i) when examined through the nostril, as in rhinoscopy, but only contain mucosa. *see also Turbinates*

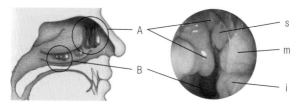

necro- (NEK-roh) death

Necrosis (neh-KROH-sihs): death of a cell, a group of cells, or a T due to disease.

neo- (NEE-oh) new

Neti pot: a small pot filled with solutions & used for nasal irrigation, to relieve flush out the nasal cavity & relieve sinusitis & nasal congestion The head is placed on the side & the pot tipped so that solution goes through the nostril & comes out the other side(1). This is then repeated. The mucus is softened & "full" sinuses often empty into the cavity(2), clearing the region.

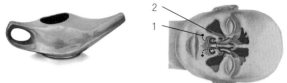

neur- nerve

Neuron (N) (NEW-ron) AKA Nerve cell: *Gk. neuron = nerve* a cell of NT characterized by its specialization to conduct impulses (conductivity) to & from its nucleus via depolarization of it CM *adj. neural. see **the A to Z of Peripheral Nerves** for more detail*

Neurotransmitter (new-roh-TRANS-mit-er): a molecule that transmits or inhibits the transmission of N impulses across synapses.

neutro- neutral

Neutrophil (NEW-troh-fil): a type of granular, phagocytic WBC characterized by a cytoplasm that stains pink/purple in a neutral stain i.e. does not preferentially take up either acid or base of the stain.

noci-(noh-SEE) pain

Non respiratory air movements (NRAM): movement of air through the RT which does not involve GE. These movements are reflexes & include: burping, coughing, crying, hiccupping laughing, talking, sneezing, whispering, yawning* *It is possible yawning does involve GE *see MT.*

Norma: *Lt. = pattern or rule, or aspect; adj. normal according to rule.*

Nose AKA Proboscis: the midline facial projection which covers the nasopharynx & acts to warm, filter & humidify inspired air.

The nasal MM lines the nasal cavity & is responsible for "smelling" – air is funneled via the turbinates to pass by this sensitive T. The loss of this sense may be indicative of a more serious pathological process.

The mucosal secretions if excessive can cause the nose to become "runny", congested &/or blocked preventing any AF. Swelling of the nasal MM, poor sinus drainage ± ↑ nasal secretions, or drying of nasal secretions can cause sinusitis see also boogey MT for discussion of other components.

Nose picking *see Rhinotillexis / Picking the nose*

Nostril AKA Naris: the opening of the nose - generally lined with hairs internally, which helps to filter large particles & moisten the incoming air. Although both openings are often symmetrical of the 2 nostrils 1 is always dominant – although which one may change. This is due to the fact that there are 2 main chemical reactions needed to smell: the fast & the slow. Hence having 2 nostrils improves olfaction, while not compromising on breathing. The reasons for the changing of the dominant nostril is not known. *see also Naris*

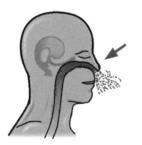
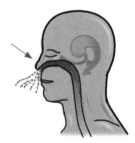

O

oc- **against in front of**

Obstructive lung disease diseases that narrow the airways & ⬆R to airflow

Occult hidden

oedem- (er-DEEM-) **swelling** **(AS edem-)**

Oedema AS Edema: pathological swelling of an organ or region

-oid **like**

olig- **scant deficient few little**

-ology (o-loh-jee) **study of**

-oma (OH-mar) tumor or lump

or- ora- *Lt. ora = margin or edge* **mouth**

Organ: a group of Ts & cells which are bound together to perform a specific function

Organelle (or-gan-EL): a component of a cell that has a consistent, similar structure in other cells & performs a particular function. For more details *see the A to Z of Major Organs*

Orifice (or-EE-fiss): an opening especially into the mouth or a cavity *see also Meatus*

ortho- (or-thoh) **straight straightening**

Oscitation: *Lt oscito = to open ones mouth* **AKA Yawning** *see also non respiratory air movements*

-osis **condition of / disease of – non-inflammatory**

oxy- (OKS-ee) **sharp**

P

Palate: a roof *adj. palatal or palatine.*

pali- **recurrence**

pan- **general overall**

Pandiculation: to yawn & stretch at the same time, common to all vertebrates at all ages. It follows patterns related to the circadian rhythm, but also is related to arousal levels. *see also Yawn*

Papilla (pap-PIHL-ah): *Lt. = nipple or teat*; a small finger-shaped projection *adj. papillary.*

par- **beside**

para- **against aside abnormal unequal**

Paralysis (PA-ral-i-sis): *Gk. para = beside, near, lyein = to loosen*; loss or impairment of muscle function.

46

Parasagittal: unequal vertical divisions b/n R & L in the body *see also Sagittal & Midsagittal*

Parasomnia: a category of sleep disorder involving abnormal behaviours, dreams, emotions & perceptions that occur while around the sleeping process. Causes are often associated with respiratory disorders e.g. sleep apnea

Parenchyma (pa-REN-kïm-ah): *Gk para = beside or near, en = in & chein = to pour* the functioning elements of an organ as opposed to the structural or supporting elements (**≠ Stroma**)

Paresis (Pa-REE-sis): *Gk. = relaxation,* but has come to mean partial paralysis.

Parietal (pa-RĬ-eh-tal): *Lt. parietalis, pertaining to paries = wall* pertaining to the outer wall of a cavity or organ i.e. parietal layer of the pleura outer of the 2 layers of the coverings of the lungs ≠ **Visceral**.

Paroxysm (PAR-roks-m) AKA Paroxysm of coughing: *Gk. para = during, oxys = acute or sharp,* a sudden violent worsening of pre-existing symptoms - a series of sharp repeated coughing in the one expiration occurring intermittently during the day with few coughs in b/n associated with **Pertussis (AKA Whooping cough)** *adj.- paroxysmal*

Pars: *Lt. = part.*

path- / -pathy   disease / disease of

Pathology (path-ol-LOH-jee): the study or science of diseases.

Pectus AKA Chest

Pectus carinatum AKA Barrel chest AKA Pigeon chest: is a breastbone (Sternum) & rib cartilage deformity that causes the chest to bow outward. It is caused by a defect in the tough CT (cartilage) that holds the ribs to the breastbone.

 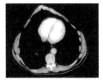

Pectus excavatum AKA Hollow chest AKA Sunken chest: often congenital ± familial it may develop at puberty where the ribs grow inward depressing the Sternum, a common symptom of the Marfan's syndrome, as with kyphoscoliosis this may interfere with respiration by not allowing for adequate thorax expansion

 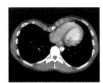

Pelvis: *Lt. = basin, adj.- pelvic.*

per-   through, excessive

Perfusion (Q): *Gk. peri = around* - the amount of BF through an organ &/T. wrt RT this is to allow for adequate GE – for the purpose of oxygenation & AB regulation in the body

peri-   around, about, beyond

Peristalsis: *Gk. peri = around & stellein - to constrict*; a circular constriction passing as a wave along a muscular tube; *adj.- peristaltic.*

Pertussis AKA Whooping cough AKA 100 day cough: *Gk per = severe tussis = cough* a highly contagious airborne bacterial In (Bordetella Pertussis). Several stages in this disease process
1 initial catarrhal stage (1-10 days); nasal congestion ↑ AR …
2 paroxysmal stage (<100 days) - weeks of violent & severe paroxysmal coughing & inspirational WHooooP; which may cause: subconjunctival Hgs, broken ribs, pneumothorax, subcutaneous emphysema & fainting.
3 convalescent stage (1-2 weeks)
Other complications include: neurological damage from anoxia or as a result of the violence of the coughing
If < 1yo where there may be no coughing reflex – so the infection may present as long periods of apnea.

Petiolus (pet-ey-OH-lus): *Lt. pes = foot* stem or stalk - usually in reference to the epiglottic petiolus see Epiglottis

phago (FAY-goh)   to eat

Phagocytosis: the active ingestion of particles, by a cell & their subsequent digestion & inactivation w/n that cell

Pharynx (FA-rinks) *Gk. pharunx = throat* space behind the nose & mouth leading to the larynx & oesophagus *see MT*

Phlegm (FLEM) AKA Sputum: *Gk. phlegma = inflammation; Lt = clammy moisture of the body* a particular form of mucus restricted to the RT & sinus secretions

Phonation (FOHN-ay-shon): is the sound resulting from the adduction of the VCs. In expiration the VCs drawn together & via suction create vibrations that emit audible sound waves(1). As the speed of the air ↑, the pressure causes the VCs to be drawn closer to each other & ↑ volume of the voice. The clarity is compromised in aspiration or whispering(2) where the VCs are not together & the sound becomes breathier. In normal inspiration the VCs are far apart(3).

 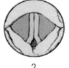

1   2   3

physi- (FIZ-ee) natural

Physiological Dead Space (PDS): the volume of gas which does not equilibrate with B. PDS = ADS + additional volume relating to alveoli which has a high V/Q ratio (>1)

"Picking the nose" AKA Rhinotillexis: colloquial term for cleaning out the entrance of the nasal cavity via a finger - & possibly consuming the dried nasal secretion **(bogies)** removed **AKA mucophagy** - which may be beneficial for the immune system by exposing it to new bacterial Ags
Note the finger usually cannot extend to the olfactory mucosa or turbinates but only to the end of the nostril

Pineal (pĭ-NEE-al) gland AKA Epithalamus: *Lt. pinea = a pine cone*
a small endocrine gland located at the posterior end of the diencephalon, forming a part of the roof of the third ventricle, see also Melatonin.

Pituitary (pit-EW-it-ar-ee) gland AKA Hypophysis: *Lt. pituita = mucous or phlegm*, the gland was thought to produce mucous which was discharged through the nose; a small, endocrine gland located inferior to the hypothalamus & attached to it by way of a short stalk.

-plasia (FAY-zee-uh) growth

Plasma (PLAZ-mah): fluid formed when B settles <u>w/o clotting</u> – clotting factors present- (as opposed to serum when the B clots & the remaining fluid is serum – clotting factors all having been used up)

pleur- (PLER) lungs respiratory

Pleura (PLEW-rah): *Gk. = a rib* but has not come to mean the serous membrane lining the lungs (visceral layer) & inner rib & intercostal surfaces (parietal layer) associated with the lungs *pl = pleurae*

Pleural effusion: fluid in the intrapleural space (b/n the 2 pleural layers)

Plexus (PLEKS-uhs) *Lt. = a network or plait.* a network of interconnecting Ns, veins, or lymphatic vessels

pneumo (NEW-moh) relating to lungs / respiratory system

Pneumoconiosis: disease of the lungs due to inhalation of FBs particles e.g. coal, dust, silicon, & other antigenic particles e.g. pollen, characterized by IF, coughing, & fibrosis *for more details see **The A to Z of Lung Failure***

Pneumocytes: the cells lining the alveoli - Type I & Type II cells, sometimes including alveolar macrophages *see MT Cells of Respiration*

Pneumonia: lung IF caused by bacterial or viral Ins; the alveoli become inflamed & fill with pus, consolidating. This may affect one or both lungs *(double pneumonia).*

Pneumotaxic centre: respiratory area of the pons which is thought to cut short inspiration

Pneumothorax: gas entering into the intrapleural space may causing lung collapse *see MT*

Polymers: repeated "monomer" units as in several monomers of the collagen fibre placed together but not enough to be a complete fibre *see also Monomers*

Polyp (PO-lip): structure with stalk and rounded, swollen head see Nasal Polyp

Polysomnography: overnight sleep studies

por- passageway

Post-nasal drip (PND) AKA post nasal drip syndrome (PNDS): is caused by the excessive mucus production by the nasal mucosa, which accumulates in the throat (back of the nose). Causes may one or more of the following: allergies, rhinitis, sinusitis, gastro-esophageal reflux disease, disorders of swallowing, or over medication of nasal medications.

postero- posterior part

Posterior (post.) (pos-TEE-ree-or): *Lt. post = behind (in place or time).* a directional term describing the location of a part being toward the back or rear side relative to another part.

prae- in front of before

pre- in front of before

pro- in front of

Process (PROH-sehs): *Lt. = going forwards, indicating growing out, i.e. an outgrowth,* general term used to describe any marked projection or prominence usually bone

proct- anus rectum

Proton: positively charged subatomic particle found in the nucleus of an atom. A term which synonymously is used for a hydrogen ion H^+ (when the electron is removed from the hydrogen atom).

Proximal (PROKS-i-mal): *Lt. proxime = nearest* a directional term indicating a body part that is located nearer to the origin or point of attachment to the trunk than another; ≠ **Distal**

pseudo- (syoo-doh) false

pulmo- lung

Pulmonary embolism (PE): thrombi lodging in the pulmonary vasculature causing V/Q mismatches of varying severity - a serious complication of venous thrombosis. *see also Embolus Thrombus*

Pulmonary fibrosis: a restrictive lung disease where the interstitium is thickened with collagen deposition - an endpoint of many lung diseases.

Pulmonary hypertension: ↑ arterial P in the lungs - due to: C.F., COAD, interstitial lung disease, OSA, recurrent PE- any process which makes it harder to push B through the normally LP pulmonary circulation

Pulmonary oedema: fluid in the lungs(3) generally secondary to ↑ P from the RV(2) after heart damage or in CCF. Pressure builds in the pulmonary circulation as the RV fails - fluid moves into the alveoli, causing damage to the cells & causing IF reaction. This results in ↑ fluid in the alveoli - stiffening the lungs & ↓ GE. The person "drowns" internally. In the short term this may resolve, but in the long term initiating the repair process ↑ fibroblast proliferation causing interstitial lung disease.

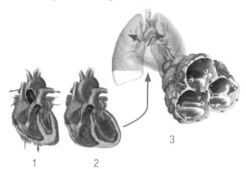

1   2   3

Non-cardiogenic or 1° pulmonary oedema results from ↑ alveolar permeability with a normal BP. Fluid flows into the alveoli & is not adequately drained, e.g. allergies, anaphylaxis, an Ag will cross the BGB cause ImR releasing immunoglobulins & ↑ fluid leakage into the alveoli *see also Allergies.*

R

Radial traction: wrt the pulmonary system is the outward pull of the lung parenchyma which "holds open" the smaller airways

Radicals: charged atomic particles or charged polyatomic groups which may be bound to larger molecules or freely disassociated & "unbound" - ***free radicals*** - refer to an unbound charged ions or molecules - they are highly reactive.

rami- (ray-mee) branch

REM-atonia: a bodily state wherein motor Ns are not stimulated & reflex signals are not relayed to the brain. Sufficient external stimulants, however, may cause a person to wake from their sleep for the purpose of sneezing, although any sneezing occurring afterwards would take place with a partially awake status at minimum.

Rapidly Acting Nerve ending: a N which has a rapidly decreasing response to a stimulus even if the response is still present

Rapidly Adapting Receptor: receptors in the airways which respond to dynamic changes in the lung volume or to irritants in the RT

Recruitment: the process in the pulmonary circulation whereby additional BVs open up & carry B when there is an ↑ in CO

Refractory period: the quiescent period following activation during which T such as N & muscle cannot be fully stimulated again

Reid index: the proportion of the total airway thickness that is made up of mucous glands. it is normally <40%

Residual volume (RV): the volume of gas that is left in the lungs at the end of maximum expiration

Respiratory Exchange Ratio AKA Respiratory Quotient: ratio of CO_2 output to O_2 input

Respiratory Tree: a name for the treelike pattern of the branching airways not including the alveoli

Restrictive Lung Diseases: diseases which stiffen the lungs (generally due to fluid) so that expansion of the lungs is compromised

retro- *prefix Lt. = backwards.* **located behind**

rhe- (REE) **flow**

rheum- (ROOM) **mucoid or watery discharge / relating to joint pain**

rhinus / rhino- (RYE-noh) **pertaining to the nose**

Rhinitis: IF of the nose this could be due to infection or due to allergy **e.g. allergic rhinitis AKA hay fever**

Rhinotillexis AKA "Picking the nose": the act of putting a digit into the nose with the object of removing dried mucoid secretions (boogies) ± eating them (**Mucophagy**); when excessive or pathological **Rhinotillexomania**

Ridge: elevated bony growth often roughened.

Rima Glottidis: structures surrounding the space (glottis) b/n the vocal cords

Rostral: directional towards the ant./front (of the brain)

rigor- *Lt rigor = stiffness*

Runny nose *see Nasal congestion*

S

Sarcoidosis (SAR-koid-oh-sis): a disease of granuloma T which may cause interstitial lung disease

Secrete (seh-KREET): *Lt. secretus = separated*; hence, to produce a chemical substance by glandular activity *adj. secretory; noun, secretion.*

semi- half partial

seps- decay

Septum: *Lt. saeptum = fenced in*; hence, a dividing fence or partition- generally of CT. wrt the RT the nasal septum – divides the nasal opening into 2 nostrils. This is uneven in a deviated septum & may interfere with breathing *see also nostril*

Serosa (ser-OH-suh) AKA Serous membrane: *Lt. = like serum, serum- like* any serous membrane. (also, the outer membranous layer of a visceral organ containing BS & NS as well as lymphatic drainage), similar to the capsule of an organ.

Shunt: going from the arterial to the venous side w/o going through the capillaries wrt RT deoxygenated B which passes from the R to the L circulation w/o becoming oxygenated, hence reducing the oxygenation of the B. This occurs in underperfused areas of the lung or in pneumonia where the alveoli become fluid filled and hence canto be ventilated

Sigh (SĪ): a deep slow inspiration & expiration, generally occurs singly *see MT non respiratory air movement*

Sinus: a space usually w/in a bone lined with MM, such as the frontal & maxillary sinuses in the head, (also, a modified BV usually vein with an enlarged lumen for blood storage & containing no or little muscle in its wall). Sinuses may contain air, blood, lymph, pus or serous fluid depending upon location & health of the subject *adj. sinusoid. see also MT*

Sinusitis: IF of the sinuses - SS headache, facial pain, feeling of head heaviness associated with nasal infections allergies. The normally air filled spaces(s) become fluid filled(si) in acute sinusitis, or permanently swollen(sw) & hypertrophied(H) in chronic sinusitis, as demonstrated in this MRI.

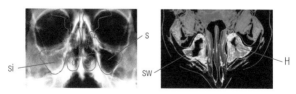

Sleep: a naturally recurring state of mind characterized by altered consciousness, ↓ motor & sensory activity, ↓ movement & awareness of surroundings. It occurs in repeating periods, & has 2 highly distinct forms - non-REM & REM sleep. During REM, there is: rapid eye movement + virtual paralysis of the of the body, quelling a number of reflexes including sneezing. Most systems are in an anabolic state, ↑ repair & regeneration of a number of systems. The internal circadian clock triggers sleepiness with the onset of darkness, via melatonin. The purpose of sleep seems to reset the body & mind to a more balanced better working condition. This may be assisted by dreaming. *see also Melatonin*

Sleep Apnea: a disorder of the respiratory system where breathing is interrupted during sleep. The main type, Obstructive Sleep Apnea (OSA) is caused by blockage of the AF due to reduced pharyngeal opening - the tongue moves posteriorly & blocks the opening. Certain sleep position predispose to this occurring. *see also MT*

Soma (SOH-mah): *Gk. = the body* pertaining to the body or the main part of an organ or a cell but not the viscera *adj. somatic*

Somite: *Gk. soma = body*, hence an embryonic body segment.

Sneeze AKA Sternutation: is a forceful convulsive expulsion of air through the nose & mouth. Generally irritation of the MM in the nose, causes a sharp inhalation(I), which is then blocked from exhalation until P is built up in the thorax, against a closed glottis, causing a sudden violent release of air(V) mainly through the nose. Sneezing is linked to other sudden changes e.g. rapid change in temperature, wind, dust, changes in light &/or Ins. The *high velocity spray of mucous* generated can lead to the spread of disease, so covering the sneeze spray is recommended(B). Sneezing cannot occur during sleep due to REM- atonia. *see also MT non respiratory air movements*

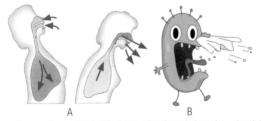

A   B

Snore: the sound associated with air escaping through the palate when it is obstructing breathing usually in inspiration *see also MT Sleep Apnea*

Snot: slang term for the mucous in the nose, mucous which "runs out of the nose"(A) or is issued from the nose in a sneeze(B). Snot contains mucopolysaccharides dissolved in water ± infective particles, as such it can be highly contagious. It varies from clear, cream, grey, yellow to green (brown if it contains B), although these colours are not indicative of its infective status, *see also Bogey*

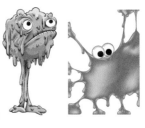

Spasm: *Gk. spasmos = an involuntary contraction of a muscle; adj. spastic, or spasmodic.*

Spasmodic dysphonia: the spasm of muscles of the larynx during speech - often due to anxiety & overuse of the voice.

Sphincter (SVINK-ter): *Gk. sphinkter = a tight binder*, i.e. a circular muscle which closes an orifice; preventing passage of material *adj. sphincteric. see also Constrictor*

Spine: a thorn descriptive of a sharp, slender process/protrusion commonly used regarding the spinous processes (SP) of the vertebral bodies *adj.- spinous see also MT bones ligs of the thorax & **The A to Z of Bones, Joints & Ligaments and the Back** for more details*

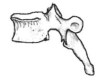

spir- coiled, respiration, breath

Spirometry: a diagnostic technique used to measure the speed of the AF & the volume exhaled from the lungs

Sputum AKA Phlegm: *Lt speuere = to spit* generally contains more saliva than phlegm which is mainly mucus, & actively coughed up

steno- narrow

Stereocilium: *Gk. stereos = solid, & cilium = eyelash*, hence a non-motile microvillus, present in the RT epithelium lower down than the ciliated epithelium.

Sternum AKA Breastbone: *Gk. sternon = chest or breast; adj. sternal.*

Stoma (STOH-mah): *Gk. = a mouth.*

Stratum *Lt. = a covering sheet, or layer.* generally referring to the skin layers pertaining to a multiple-layered arrangement *adj. stratified*

Stroma (STROH-mah): *Gk. = bed or mattress* supporting bed of cells, CT or matrix upon which the parenchyma builds *see also Parenchyma*

sub- under / less than / partial

suf-   under

super-   over

Superficial (supf.) (soo-per-FISH-al): *Lt. super = above & facies = surface*; hence, nearer the surface. A directional term indicating the location of a part that is toward or nearer to the body surface relative to another ≠ **Deep.**

Superior (soo-PEER-ee-or) AKA Craniad AKA Cephalad: *Lt. superus = above* a directional term indicating the location of a part that is nearer to the head region than another.

supra- *Lt. prefix = superior* **to above over**

Surface Tension (St): Forces of attraction b/n liquid molecules are 3 dimensional(A) but on the surface(B) the same forces are dispersed over 2 dimensions only & so are much stronger. This means it requires more force to ↑ the SA in inspiration, unless there are molecules to disperse these attractive forces such as those of the surfactant proteins (SP).

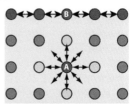

Surfactant: a lipid-protein complex which stabilizes respiratory units involved in GE by lining the walls & ↓ St. It also acts to protect the lungs from inhaled pathogens. Surfactant is rich in phospholipids 75% (mainly DPPC)(L) & apoproteins 10%(Sp). Other components include carbohydrates 2%(CHO) & neutral fats - mainly cholesterol 13%(F). Surfactant is secreted by Clara cells & Type II alveolar cells, which release the substance via lamellar bodies. Type II cells reabsorb the material & reuse it, with respiration. Macrophages(M) mop up degraded/oxidized surfactant(Sd). Surfactant is degraded by air pollutants including: asbestos, silica & tobacco smoke.

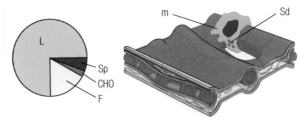

Surfactant proteins (Sp): Sp B & C are the 2 major proteins of surfactant, helping to unpack the EC lamellar bodies(LB), after they are extruded from the CM. St-stabilizing lipid membranes are formed in the air-water(AW) interface of the alveolar surface. These Sps insert & remove the DPPC & other lipids into & out of the covering membrane as the SA changes with respiration, keeping the film stable while maintaining a low St.

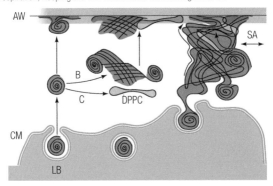

sym- together union association

Symphysis (SIM-fis-sis): *Gk. syn = with & physis = growth*; a joint - bone + fibrocartilage + bone generally used for joints in the median plane, often fuse later in life

syn- the close proximity of, or fusion of 2 structures

Synchondrosis (sin-KRON-droh-sis): *Gk. syn = with, & chondros = cartilage*; a joint - bone + cartilage + bone as in the rib cage

Syndrome (sin-DROHM): *Gk. syn = with, & dromos = running*; i.e. a group of SS, characteristic of a certain pathology.

T

tect- covering

terti (ter-shi-) third

Throat (THROHT): common term for pharynx ± the larynx particularly in a *sore throat* or *clearing the throat* - either when mucus moved up from the upper RT reaches the VCs from below or particles fall on the VCs from above triggering the gag reflex causing them to be expelled or swallowed,.

Thrombus: a B clot(B) that has formed in a vein or artery(a), often assoc with atheromatous plaques(p), which interrupts or blocks BF. These may break off & travel in the vascular system before impacting in the lumens of small

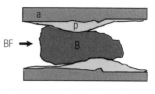

BVs. If in thesystemic arterial system - this means that they will impact in arteries of the pulmonary circulation - pulmonary emboli *see also Emboli.*

Thyroid: *Gk. thyreos = shield, & eidos = shape or form*; shaped like a shield (shields the glottis).

Tissue (T) (TI-shoo): a group of similar cells that combine to form a common function.

Tongue (tung): the muscular organ anchored to the floor of the mouth & walls of the pharynx. It plays major roles in swallowing & speech formation. Posterior movement of the tongue plays a role in sleep apnea *see MT*

Tonsil (TON-sil): *Lt. = little pole* a small organ of lymphoid T consisting of aggregations of fixed lymphocytes & CT embedded in a MM. The opening of the pharynx is ringed with tonsils, the main ones being: the palatine tonsil(1) - around the soft palate , the pharyngeal tonsil(2) in the oropharyngeal walls & the lingual tonsil(3) - at the root of the tongue. They all have both diffuse (d) & nodular (n) lymphoid tissue. Tonsils may trap particles in their crypts (c) & this can cause IF & tonsil stones. *see also MT throat*

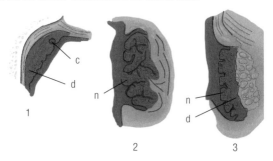

Tonsil stones: dead cells, debris, & bacteria which get trapped in the nook & crannies of the tonsils & then harden into calcified pockets. The stones are mainly white & contain calcium.

Trachea (TRAK-ee-uh): rough

Transverse AKA Horizontal: directional term to go across

Tuberosity: a large rounded process or eminence, a swelling or large rough prominence often associated with a tendon or ligament attachment.

Turbinate: a child's spinning top, hence shaped like a top; an old term for the nasal conchae. The inferior turbinate(i) is a separate bone & can be reduced as it can enlarge obstructing nasal breathing(io).

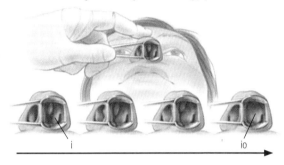

Trauma (TRAW-mah): *Gk injury,* wound physical or psychological

tri- three

troph- (TROHF) nutrition

Tunica (TEW-nik-uh): *Lt. = shirt; hence a covering.*

Tussive: of or related to coughing – hence anti-tussives are used to suppress coughing

U

Ulcer (UL-ser) *Lt ulcus = wound, sore,* hence lack of continuity on the epidermis - must penetrate all the layers of the skin or MM.

uni- first one

Uvula (YOUV-you-luh): *Lt = little grape* - c.f. the dangling tissue seen in the back of the throat - extension of the soft palate *see MT*

V

vaso- pertaining to BF

Vallecula: *see Epiglittis*

Vascular (VAS-kyew-lar): *Lt. vasculum, diminutive of vas; hence,* pertaining or containing BVs.

Vein (vayn): a BV that transports B from body Ts to the heart. *adj. venous*

ven- vein

Venipuncture (VEEN-EE–punc-tewr): puncturing of a vein – (in order to take a B sample)

Venter: *Lt. = belly*; hence, ventral, pertaining to the belly side. *adj. ventral*

Ventilation: aeration with gas wrt air in the pulmonary system suitable for GE

Ventilation / Perfusion (V/Q): ratio should be 1 so there is a matching in the circulation & aeration e.g. pneumonia < 1 / emphysema > 1

Ventral: a directional term describing the location of a part nearer to the anterior or front side of the body relative to another.

vesic- to do with the bladder

Vertebra: turning point *pl vertebae*

Vesicle (VEEZ-ik-el): *diminutive of Lt. vesica = bladder, hence a little bladder* any membrane enclosed bubble w/n a cell - generally with the same bilipid layered as the CM. It is possible for the vesicle to generate a separate internal environment w/n the cell - the cell's organelles are forms of vesicles see also Organelle. *see the A to Z of Major Organs for more details*

Vestibule (VEHS-tih-byewl): *Lt. vestibulum = entrance hall* a small space that opens into a larger cavity or canal. A vestibule is found in the inner ear, mouth, nose & vagina.

Visceral (VIHS-er-ahl): *Lt. viscus = an internal organ* pertaining to the internal components (mainly the organs) of a body cavity; pertaining to the outer surface of an internal organ (≠ **Parietal**).

Viscus: *Lt. = an internal organ, pl. - viscera, adj.- visceral.*

Vital: *Lt. vita = life.*

vivi- alive

Voice AKA Human voice: consists of sounds made using the vocal folds. It is used for talking, singing, laughing, crying, screaming etc. The human voice is specifically a part of human sound production in which the vocal folds are the primary sound source. Hence it does not include all forms of phonation e.g. whispering *see also MT*

Voice loss AKA Laryngitis: IF on the vocal cords or surrounding T in the larynx will often result in loss of the voice, partially or completely. By changing the tone of the muscles or the shape of the T folds through which air passes, the voice can be permanently or temporarily lost or changed. *see also Phonation*

volv- turn

Vulgar: *Lt vulgaris = usual*; common, plentiful

W

Wheeze: the whistling sound made on expiration when there is additional AR,

X

xen- (ZEN) different
xero- (ZAIR-oh) dry
Xerostoma: dry mouth

Y

Yawn/ing: *from old English* **AKA Oscitation** a reflex contraction, lasting about 6s, mainly of the Medial Pterygoid muscle with a simultaneous inhalation of air & stretching of the eardrums, followed by an exhalation, & may occur in clusters. Different riggers include: sleepiness, boredom, stress, P changes (i.e. in an aeroplane), when there is low Oxygen levels, & in a warm room. Seeing others yawn will also trigger yawning. *One yawn produces several good yawners.*
Paradoxically it may be a device to make a person more alert & is associated with reflex tearing. The sharp inspiration of the yawn may cause the brain temperature to drop slightly (0.1C°) & so increase its activity. It is possible it also stretches the throat muscles & may help prevent loss of tone in this area, but in most situations to yawn is considered rude & antisocial. *see also Pandiculation, MT*

Z

-zyme enzyme

Anatomical Planes & Positions

A = Anterior Aspect from the front = or / Posterior Aspect from the back.
Used interchangeably with ventral and dorsal respectively
B = Lateral Aspect from either side
C = Transverse / Horizontal plane
D = Midsagittal plane = Median plane; trunk moving away from this
plane = lateral flexion or lateral movement
plane medial movement;
limbs moving away from this direction = abduction
limbs moving closer to this plane = adduction
Note parasagittal plane / sagittal plane - indicates planes in the
same direction but other than in the middle
E = Coronal plane
F = Median

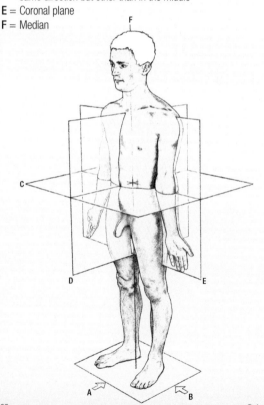

© A. L. Neill

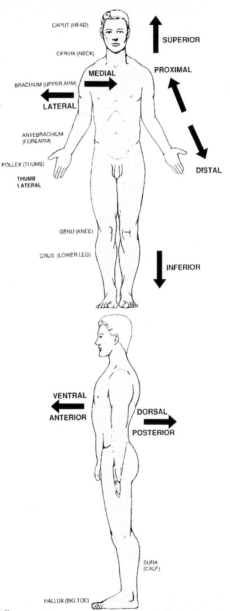

CAPUT (HEAD)

CERVIX (NECK)

SUPERIOR

PROXIMAL

MEDIAL

BRACHIUM (UPPER ARM)

LATERAL

ANTEBRACHIUM
(FOREARM)

POLLEX (THUMB)

THUMB
LATERAL

DISTAL

GENU (KNEE)

CRUS (LOWER LEG)

INFERIOR

VENTRAL

ANTERIOR

DORSAL

POSTERIOR

SURA
(CALF)

HALLUX (BIG TOE)

© A. L. Neill

The Cells of the Respiratory Tract

The following images are diagrams of isolated specialized cells of the RT, including the major cell types involved in allergic reactions such as asthma hay fever & other atopies.

1 olfactory basal cell

2 olfactory gland cell - dark cell

3 olfactory gland cell - light cell

4 olfactory sensory cell

5 olfactory sustenacular cell AKA columnar epithelial support cell

---

6 mesothelial cells

---

7 alveolar lining cell - type I

8 alveolar secretory cell - type II

9 alveolar macrophage

10 brush cell

11 reticular cell

---

12 basal epithelial cell

13 ciliated epithelial cell

14 goblet cell AKA mucus secreting cell

15 mesenchymal cell

16 smooth muscle cells

---

17 eosinophil AKA eosinophilic leukocyte

18 mast cell

19 plasma cell

20 basophil AKA basophilic leukocyte

Image Key

	Axons / N processes
	BGB-fused BMs of vasc. endo & alveolar epi.
	BM under every epithelium
	Cilia & their basal bodies
	Eosinophilic granules
	ER - rough & smooth
	Contractile filaments Actin - lighter green Myosin - darker green
	Aveolar interstitial T full of elastic fibres
	GA
	Mucoid/lipid droplets
	Lysosomes - full of enzymes & cell debris
	NM with pores and attached ribosome
	mv with & w/o contractile filaments
	mucus (glycoprotein & mucopolysaccaride) secretions in vesicles & on surfaces
	Mitochondria with internal cristae from internal mem.
	Nuclear material inactve - mauve active - darker (also nucleolar)
	Protein deposits & secretions - including enzymes & surfactant proteins

Cells of the olfactory mucosa (1-5) include the olfactory (Bowman's) gland cells, which secrete both protein serous secretions (dark cells -2) & mucus secretions (light cells -3). Because of the high volume & extreme exposure to dry & "dirty" air in the nose, olfactory mucosal cells must be more protective against infections & moisturize better than other areas of the RT. The sustentacular(5) & glandular secretions differ from the rest of the RT. The olfactory glands secrete a continuous faster flowing & more "watery" mucus via different AQPs, than the rest of the RT. The nasal mucus (phlegm) has strong antibacterial properties, rendering a lot of the airborne bacteria harmless. The cilia of the sensory cells(4) must be able to detect & discriminate b/n various *odiferous* molecules. This generally means the molecules must be dissolved in either an aqueous (from dark cells) or lipid (from light cells) solution.

Olfactory basal cells(1) divide constantly replacing the simple columnar olfactory epithelium, which appears to be stratified - i.e. pseudo-stratified ciliated columnar epithelium (PSCCE). They also actively support the sensory axons, enclosing them in their cytoplasm.

Resident in the submucosa are mast (18) & plasma (19) cells, which when exposed to allergens, cause ↑ mucus secretions, swelling of the mucosa, sneezing & other SS of allergic rhinitis. The sinuses are lined with the same T so with additional secretions sinus drainage may be blocked causing IF (sinusitis).

Cells of the nasal vestibule & oral cavity are stratified squamous epithelium.

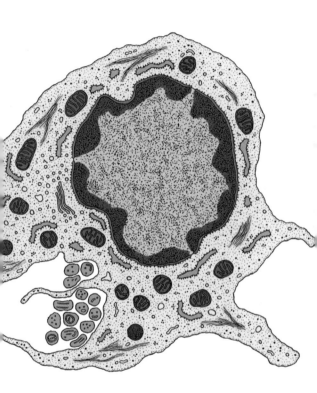

2. Olfactory gland cell - dark cell

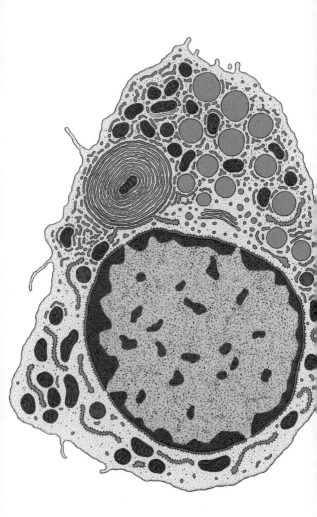

© A. L. Neill

3. Olfactory gland cell - light cell

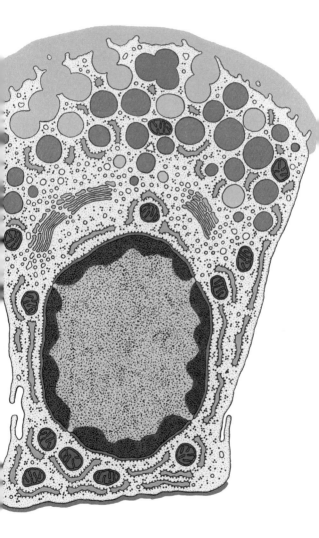

4. Olfactory sensory cell

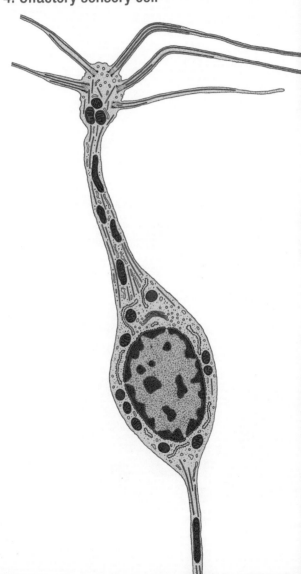

© A. L. Neill

5. Olfactory sustenacular cell
AKA columnar epithelial support cell

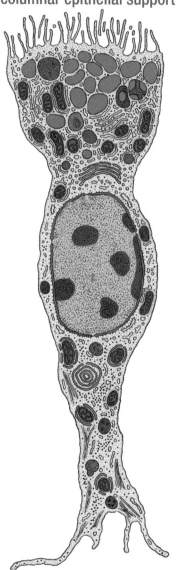

Cells of the pleura (6) Mesothelial cells form the outer flattened layers of the pleura. These squamous epithelial derived cells are phagocytic. Their many mv create a large surface area allowing them to pinocytose fluid from the pleural cavity, which contains up to 100mLs/lung & particles from the lung cavities within the alveoli. They create a smooth surface b/n the 2 layers, allowing the lungs to move over the chest wall w/o R.

6. Mesothelial cells

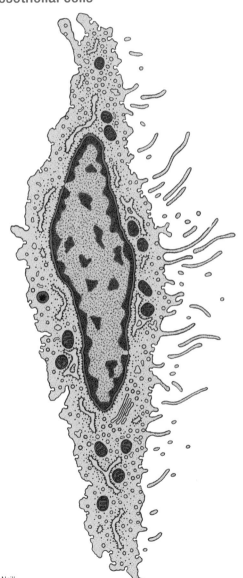

Cells of the lower RT (7-11) are involved in the GE & fluid transport. The extensive alveolar surface (~140m^2) is covered (>93%) by the Type I pneumocytes (7) which are large (>40μm in diameter) thin flattened (.1-.2μm) epithelial cells spreading over the 300 million alveoli. They share their BM with that of the respiratory capillary endothelium; each alveolus being serviced by 1000 capillary segments, forming the thin BGB (.3-.5μm). Their CMs also transport fluid rapidly via specific AQPs. The alveolar surface is covered with SPs produced in membrane bound bodies by the Type II pneumocytes(8). SPs ↓ ST which keeps the alveoli "open" & allow the gases to dissolve for GE. Type II cells also produce antiprotease enzymes mainly **α-antitrypsin** & various cytokines. They are small cuboidal cells (8-10μm) which sit in the corners of the alveoli & replace damaged Type I cells.

Dust cells or wandering alveolar macrophages (9) AKA Type III cells move b/n the alveoli via their pores & eat up any particulate matter or infectious agents.

Further up the respiratory tree & even occasionally in the alveolar ducts the flattened cells become more cuboidal & develop mv - brush cells(10). The mv may move mucus secretions away from the alveoli assisting the cilia & may phagocytose particles & drying secretions. These cells do not participate in GE, or fluid transport but they may repair damaged epithelium. The CT of the walls of bronchioles & alveoli contain large amounts of elastic fibres supported by the reticular cells(11).

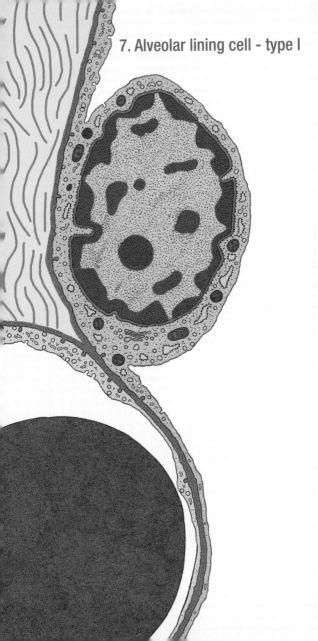

7. Alveolar lining cell - type I

8. Alveolar secretory cell - type II

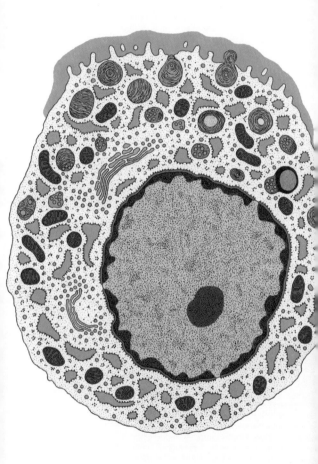

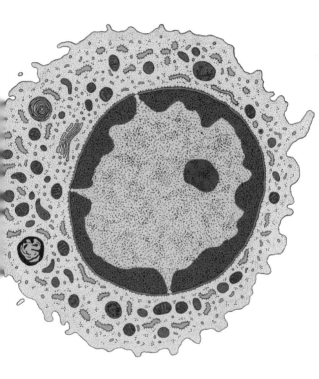

10. Brush cell

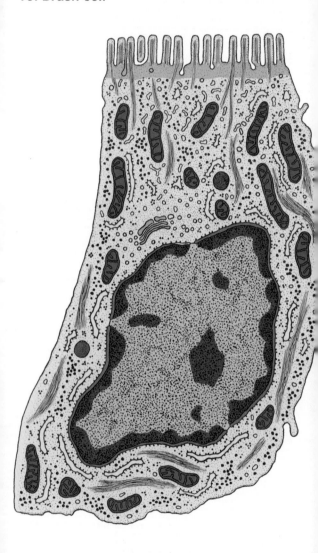

© A. L. Neill

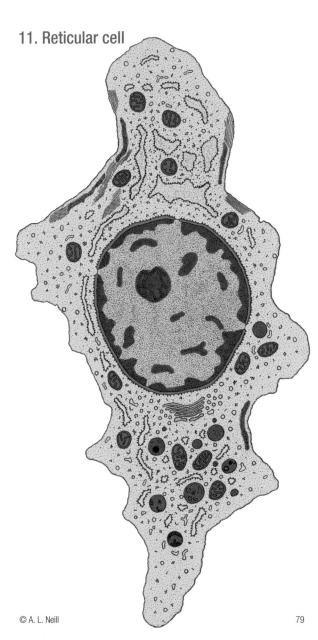

Cells of the upper RT (12-16) line the bronchi & bronchioles as PSCCE. All cells are in touch with the BM but are pushed so closely together that they appeared multilayered.

B/n the ciliated cells(13) & the goblet cells(14) which keep the surface sticky, wet & mobile are the basal cells(12) which maintain the respiratory epithelium. The sticky mucosal surface of the upper RT traps particles, sweeping them up to the VC via cilia - **mucociliated transport** - triggering the gag reflex, & causing their expulsion via coughing or swallowing *"clearing the throat"* where the mucus moves over the epiglottis & into the oesophagus.

Note that the goblet cells (14) produce the same mucopolysaccharides as the submucosal glands & are normally in a ratio of 1:5 with the ciliated cells (13). The ciliated cells have approx. 200cilia/cell. Each cilium is about 6μm tall & can beat approx. 1000-1500X/min, in tandem with each other & the other ciliated cells, allowing them to move quite large particles (b/n 9-2μm) up the RT, at 10-20mm/min.

Mesenchymal CT cells(15) support the large numbers of elastic fibres.

The smooth muscle cells(16), are often multinucleate, & act as a syncytium contracting as a unit when stimulated. Their contraction ↓ AF by ↓ the airway lumens, & can completely close off the bronchioles - where there is no cartilage.

Resident basophils (20), mast cells (18), & plasma cells (19) exposed to allergens, release IC enzymes & Abs respectively stimulating the mucus glands & smooth muscle cells, & stimulating eosinophils (17) to accumulate in the Ts.

Eosinophils release their IC granules causing thickening of the bronchiolar walls, ↑ mucus production & further eosinophilic infiltration.

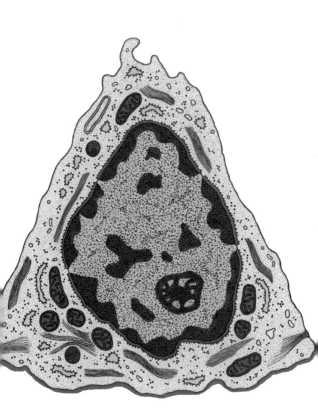

13. Ciliated epithelial cell

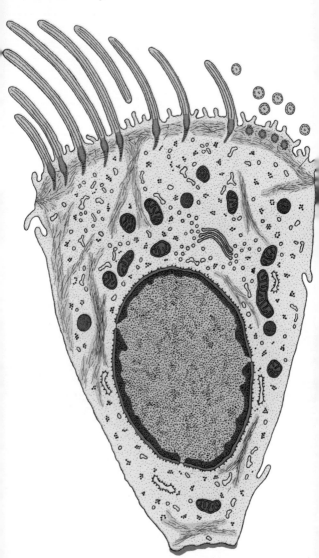

© A. L. Neill

14. Goblet cell AKA mucus secreting cell

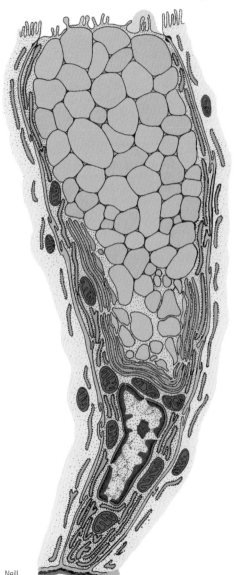

15. Mesenchymal cell

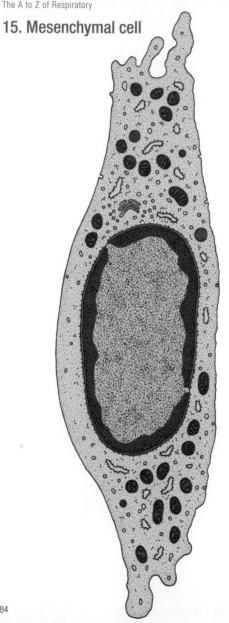

© A. L. Neill

16. Smooth muscle cells

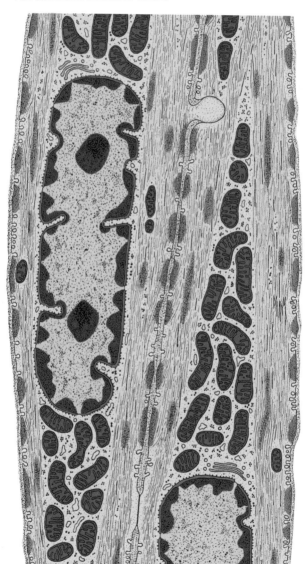

17. Eosinophil AKA eosinophilic leukocyte

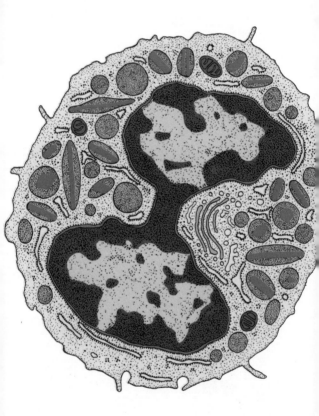

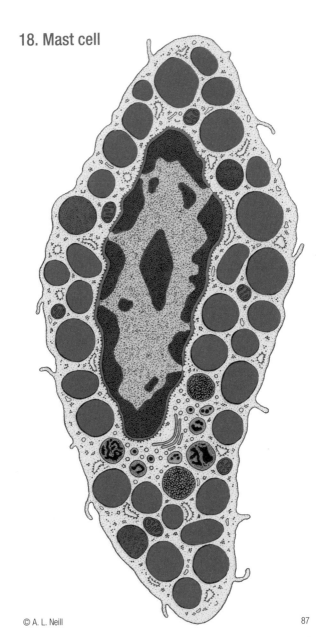

© A. L. Neill

19. Plasma cell

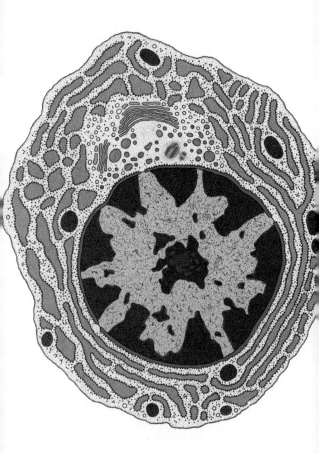

© A. L. Neill

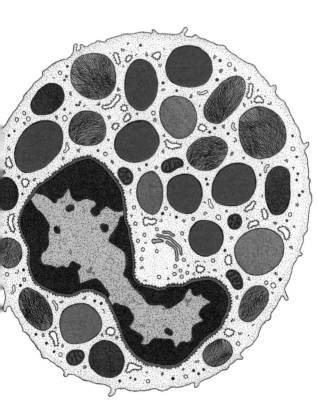

Blood gases - Acid / Base (AB) balance normal values

The lungs & kidneys regulate the AB status of the body.

Decreased CO_2 or increased HCO_3 levels create an excessive alkaline state - ALKALOSIS.

Increased CO_2 or decreased HCO_3 levels create an excessive acidotic state - ACIDOSIS.

Modality	Normal range	Comment
pH	7.35 - 7.45	<7.35 = acidosis >7.45 = alkalosis
PaO_2	75 - 100 mm Hg	O_2 pressure in normal air
$PaCO_2$	35 - 45 mm Hg	CO_2 pressure on normal air/ normal breathing In hyperventilation $PaCO_2$ falls to <35mmHg In hypoventilation PO_2 rises to <50mmHg
SaO_2	94 - 100%	Saturation of arteriolar Hb
HCO_3	22 -26 mEq/L	Bicarbonate - metabolic indicator of kidneys' role in maintaining normal pH values
CO_2	19 - 24 mEq/L	Dissolved CO_2 in blood Note O_2 is 40x less soluble than CO_2 and hence is not carried in the B
Base excess	-2 to 2 mEq/L	A positive base excess value indicates acidosis. A lower base excess value inidcates alkalosis

	Respiratory Acidosis	Respiratory Alkalosis
Causes	↑ B $[CO_2]$	↓ B $[CO_2]$
Lung conditions	emphysema COPD, severe asthma, airway obstruction	hyperventilation secondary to disease +/- altitude which causes ↓ B $[O_2]$
Other conditions	Obesity hypoventilation syndrome, excessive fatigue of the diaphragm or muscles of the rib cage, severe deformities of the rib cage or spine	
Symptoms:	Confusion ± Light-headedness secondary to hypotension Easy fatigue/lethargy Chronic cough Shortness of breath Wheezing	Confusion ± Light-headedness Fainting Muscle twitching Hand tremor / tetany Nausea, vomiting Numbness or tingling in the face ± extremities Arrhythmias 2º to electrolyte inbalance

	Common Causes	Type	pH
Respiratory Acidosis	Asphyxia Respiratory depression	Uncompensated	Decreased
	CNS depression	Compensated	Slight decrease in normal
Respiratory Alkalosis	Hyperventilation / Anxiety	Uncompensated	Increased
	Pulmonary emboli	Compensated	Slight decrease in normal
Metabolic Acidosis	Diarrhea or Renal failure	Uncompensated	Decreased
Metabolic Alkalosis	Salicylate overdose	Compensated	Slight decrease in normal
	Hypercalcemia	Uncompensated	Increased
	Antacid overdose	Compensated	Slight decrease in normal

PCO₂	HCO₃	Compensation
Increased	Increased or normal	**Ky does the following** HCO_3 - absorbed H^+ - secreted pH - ↑
Increased	Increased	
Decreased	Decreased or normal	**Ky does the following** HCO_3 - secreted H^+ - absorbed pH - ↓
Decreased	Decreased	
Decreased or normal	Decreased	**Lung / breathing compensation** Respiratory rate - ↑ CO_2 - is blown off **Ky does the following** HCO_3 - is resorbed pH - ↑
Decreased	Decreased	**Lung / breathing compensation** Respiratory rate - ↓ CO_2 - is retained **Ky does the following** H^+ - resorbed HCO_3 - secreted pH - ↓
Increased	Increased or normal	
Increased	Increased	

Table of Breathing Patterns

Type	Description
Agonal gasps	Intermittent irregular gasps
Apnoeustic	Prolonged inspiration which is held "fish breathing"
Ataxic respirations	Irregular respirations in depth, duration
Biot respirations	Irregular respirations, characterised by short shallow paroxysms followed by periods of apnoea
Bradypnoea	Deep, unusually slow breathing
Central neurogenic hyperventilation	Tachypnoeic hyperventilation- rapid deep respirations
Cheyne-Stokes respirations	Crescendo-decrescendo breathing + apnoea b/n each cycle
Eupnoea	Normal respiration
Hyperpnoea	Unusually deep breathing – but not necessarily ↑ rate only depth
Hypopnoea	Unusually shallow breathing
Kussmaul respirations	Tachypnoeic hyperventilation- rapid deep respirations
Sighing AKA Single Deep Breath	Periodic deep slow breath (>2X)
Tachypnoea	Rapid breathing , generally shallow - not hyperventilation

Pathophysiology

Representative of a neurological deficit in a dying patient.
A pulseless patient may still have occasional agonal gasps

Represents severe brain ly – in partic of the apnoeustic centre in the lower pons. This area stimulates the inspiratory Ns. Normally stretch receptors of the IC muscles will limit the extent of the inspiration

Indicative of severe brain ly or brain stem herniation

Indicative of severe brain ly, brain stem herniation or damage to the pons as in strokes or trauma. It may also occur with opioid use

Associated with sedative, narcotic &/or alcohol use, obesity, COAD, asthma, hypothyroidism, age, obstruction, brain metastases & lung cancer, ↑ intracranial P, DM ketoacidosis, drowning , diaphragmatic paralysis

↑ intracranial P, direct brain ly,
Results in respiratory alkalosis- due to low B[CO_2] levels

Unless grossly exaggerated this is not considered serious – but can be related to brain trauma & shock

2° to chemical, neurologic disorders – i.e. medications, & overdoses

A response to metabolic acidosis - ↑ acetone in the body (c.f. DM)
Results in respiratory alkalosis- due to blowing off the CO_2 - & lowering B[CO_2] levels with DM patients have a characteristic sweet breath + dry cracked lips

Forces open the alveoli – partic the lower under-ventilated sections of the lung, occurs several times in the day

This does not lower B[CO_2] – as the volumes are low – this term only relates to the rate not depth of breathing – patients may be hypoventilating

Breathing - Air & Chest Movement

Anterior view of lungs & diaphragm

Lateral view of thoracic cage, lungs & diaphragm

A - Inhaling

B - Exhaling

Inhaling sucks the air in by creating a vacuum when the ribs move up (upper ribs) & out (lower ribs) and the diaphragm contracts & flattens anchored by the 2 lowest ribs.

1 trachea
2 lungs
3 diaphragm
4 rib cage
5 Sternum
6 mouth - oral cavity
7 nasal cavity
8 pharynx
9 thorax (above the diaphragm)
10 abdomen (below the diaphragm)
11 anchoring ribs 11 & 12 do not move in respiration

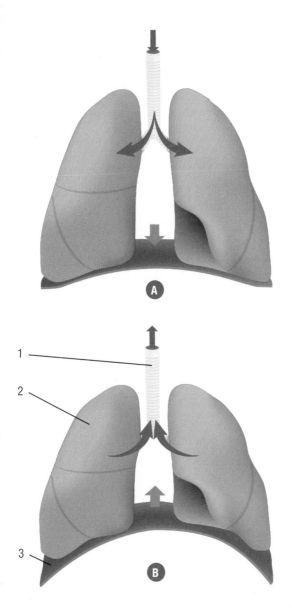

1

2

3

A

B

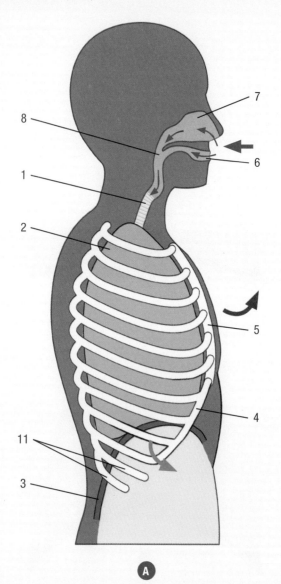

A

© A. L. Neill

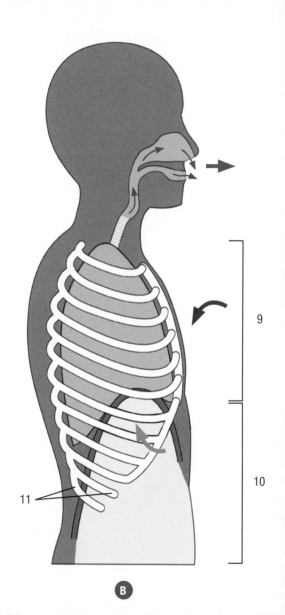

© A. L. Neill

Table of Non Respiratory Air movements (NRAM)

NRAM	Trigger
Coughing	Particles on the carina – Coughing reflex Particles on the laryngeal folds - Gag reflex Irritation of the recurrent laryngeal N – e.g. if stretched as in aortic aneurysm - *Infections can cause this pattern e.g. the common cold / influenza part of the IR/IF* medications
Crying	Sadness Allergy Emotional catharsis
Hiccupping	Reflex arc
Laughing	Amusement Happiness
Sneezing	Irritation in the upper airways Including the allergic reaction
Vocalization/ speech / phonation	Communication
Whispering	Wanting to quietly communicate Damaged VCs
Yawning	Contagion Boredom Stress Brain hot

Process	Function / *Pathophysiology*
deep inspiration closed glottis P ⬆ behind glottis glottis opened sudden rush of air out, mainly through the mouth / in severe cases also into the nasal cavity	Clears RT lower > upper IR / IF response to infection adverse drug reaction
deep inspiration slow interrupted release in expiration via opening & closing the glottis	Clears nasolacrimal duct *⬆ secretions in response to irritation* *in the eye/nose region as part of* *the IR*
diaphragm contracts spasmodically against a closed glottis – causing short irregular expirations & characteristic "HIK"	Resetting of the diaphragm respiratory cycle *Phrenic N irritation* *2° to IF in the region as in MI,* *gastric reflux, intubation*
deep inspiration slow interrupted release in expiration	Increases the abdominal P
deep inspiration closed glottis P ⬆ behind glottis glottis opened / uvula depressed sudden rush into the nasal cavity	Clears the URT
controlled expiration through the VCs, after they have orientated themselves to a partic angle – determining the pitch – the rate determines the volume	Communication *see also Larynx*
controlled expiration through the larynx, w/o involvement of the VCs – air turbulence in the larynx rather than true phonation	Quiet communication w/o VCs Alternative form of "phonation" due to damaged VCs
long deep inspiration acme / holding of breathe slow expiration (may be associated with stretching – Pandiculation)	Exercise of the throat muscles, Cooling of the brain (0.1°), ⬆ alertness, Part of a social cohesion

Circulation - overview

Schema of the systemic & pulmonary circulations & lymphatics

The body has 2 main circulations :
PULMONARY circulation; low pressure BF from the RV -
Deoxygenated B enters the RA → RV → pulmonary trunks & then goes to the lungs, where it is oxygenated then it returns to the heart (LA).
SYSTEMIC circulation; high pressure BF from the LV -
Oxygenated B enters the LA → LV → aorta & then is pushed around the body; returns to the heart deoxygenated (RA).

Arteries are defined as vessels taking B away from the heart
Veins as vessels bringing B to the heart
& lymphatics as returning extra vascular fluid to the heart
Simultaneously all 3 components are moving fluid or B around the body in their defined pathways.

	wall thickness	O_2/CO_2 levels	intravascular pressure
pulmonary arteries	++	<1 - **deoxygenated**	+/-
pulmonary veins	++	>1 - **oxygenated**	+
systemic arteries	+++++	>1 - **oxygenated**	+++++
systemic veins	++	<1 - **deoxygenated**	+++
lymphatics	+	NA	+/-

1   **RA ... →**
2   **RV ... →**
3   **R & L pulmonary arteries ... →**
4   **pulmonary capillary beds**
4A **lymphatic capillary beds**
5   **pulmonary veins**
5A **pulmonary lymphatic vessels**
5B **pulmonary LNs**
5C **lymphatic valves**
6   **LA**
6A **lymphatic duct**
7   **LV**
8   **aorta**
9   **systemic arteries**
10 **systemic capillary beds**
10A **lymphatic capillary beds**
11 **systemic veins**
11A **systemic lymphatic vessels**
11B **systemic LNs**
11C **systemic lymphatic valves**
12 **IVC / SVC**
12A **systemic lymphatic drainage ducts**

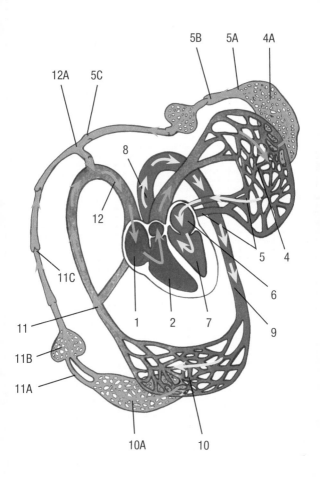

Circulation - overview

Schema of the systemic (+ portal) & pulmonary circulations

The body has 2 main circulations :

PULMONARY circulation; LP BF from the RV -(thin walled compared to the LV)

Deoxygenated B enters the RA ➔ RV ➔ pulmonary trunks & then goes to the lungs, where it is oxygenated then it returns to the heart (LA).

SYSTEMIC circulation; high pressure BF from the LV -

Oxygenated B enters the LA ➔ LV ➔ aorta & then is pushed around the body; returns to the heart deoxygenated (RA).

W/n the systemic circulation is a LP portal system, which drains the GIT.

Arteries are defined as vessels taking B away from the heart

Veins as vessels bringing B to the heart

1 **RA ➔**
2 **RV ➔**
3 **pulmonary a (L&R) ➔**
4 **pulmonary capillary beds ➔**
5 **pulmonary v(L&R) ➔**
6 **LA ➔**
7 **LV ➔**
8 **aorta ➔**
9 **coeliac trunk**
      g = L gastric a
      h = common hepatic a
      L = splenic a
      s = sinusoids of the liver (LP)
10 **superior mesenteric a**
11 **inferior mesenteric a**
12 **common iliac A&V**
13 **internal iliac A&V**
14 **external iliac A&V**
15 **systemic capillaries of the pelvis & lower limbs**
16 **arterioles & venules of the pelvis (A&V)**
17 **arterioles & venules of the lower limb (A&V)**
18 **porta hepatis AKA portal vein - LP BF**
19 **vena cavae**
      i = inferior
      s = superior
20 **BVs of the Head & Neck and upper limb**
      a = arterioles ➔
      c = capillaries ➔
      v = venules ➔

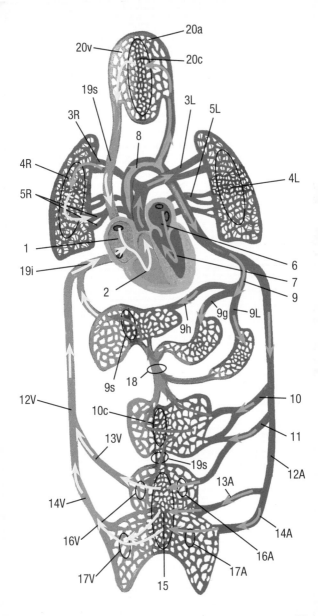

Sleep Apnea - Structural changes

Diagrams of Oral cavity & Pharynx- supine

A - normal open airway

B - obstructed airway

Obstructive sleep apnea (OSA) is when the contents of the mouth & throat relax or move to block the airway. It is often associated with snoring, and gasps or choking sounds as the brain stimulates a tightening of the throat muscles to restore airflow. It occurs most commonly in the supine position.

1 **nasal cavity**

2 **lips**
> **L = lower / u = upper**

3 **oral cavity - mouth**

4 **tongue**

5 **epiglottis**

6 **Hyoid b**

7 **palate**
> **h = hard / s = soft**

8 **eustacian tube**

9 **lingual tonsil**

10 **uvula**

11 **tubal tonsil AKA pharyngeal tonsil**

12 **palatine arches**

13 **fold of buccal mucosa**

14 **palatine tonsil AKA adenoids**

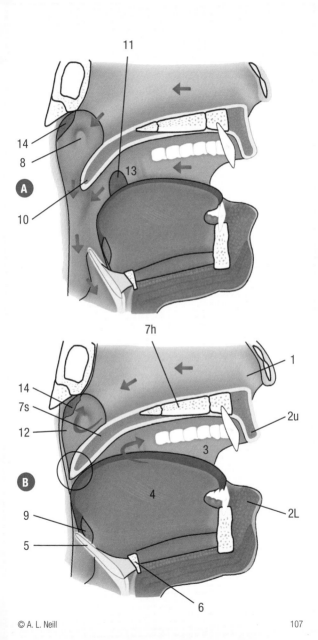

Swallowing - process

Schematic   A - initiation of swallowing

B - completion of swallowing

A food bolus is moved to the back of the throat via the tongue initiating the swallowing reflex & stopping respiration.

The pharyngeal muscles, Hyoid and soft palette are raised.

The soft palette closes off the Nasopharynx moving the food onto the vallecula of the epiglottis.

The epiglottis is pushed posteriorly closing the trachea.

The food bolus passes into the oesophagus & the Hyoid is lowered & nasopharynx opened.

The epiglottis "bounces back" anteriorly opening the trachea.

1   oral cavity = mouth
2   tongue
3   Hyoid bone
4   tracheal passage
5   oesophageal cavity
6   epiglottis v = vallecula
7   oropharynx
8   food bolus
9   soft palate
10 nasopharynx
11 Hard Palate
12 nasal cavity
13 closure of the Nasopharynx
14 closure of the Tracheal passage

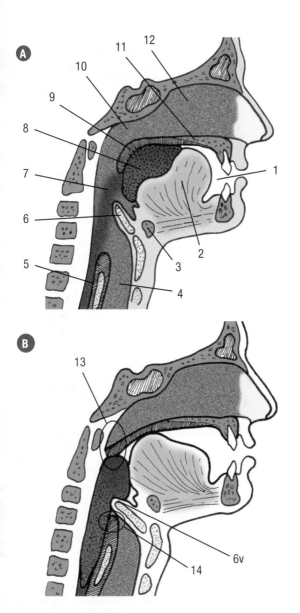

Alveoli

3 Dimensional Schema

Alveoli form tetrahedral/
cuboid shapes & are
coated with SPs which
reduce the ST & allow for
the maximum SA for GE.

1 **fused BM b/n epi
   & endo cells**
2 **lymphatic**
3 **capillary**
4 **elastic fibre**
5 **reticular fibre**
6 **type I cells -
   alveolar epi**
7 **type II cells -
   produces SPs**
8 **macrophage i =
   in the septum /
   ii = moving into
   the alveoli / iii =
   in the alveoli AKA
   Type III cell**
9 **alveolar septum**
10 **alveolar pore -
   connecting alveoli
   AKA pores of
   Kohn**

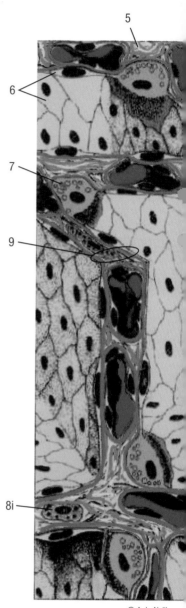

110

© A. L. Neill

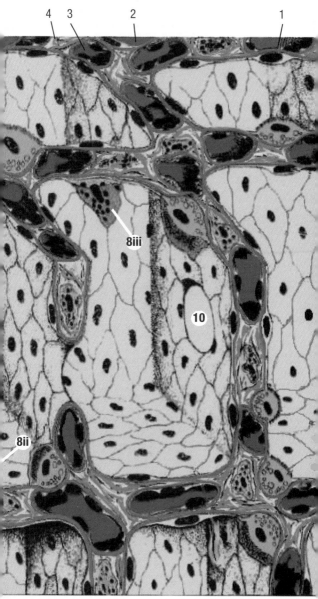

Alveoli - Blood Supply

Schema of the BS of the alveoli & lower respiratory tract site of GE

The alveoli are the site of O_2 / CO_2 exchange, as well as the respiratory acid / base balance. The BF is from the right side of the heart, bringing deoxygenated arterial B to the alveoli & taking oxygenated venous B back to the L side of the heart. B/n the RBCs & the "air" - the Blood-Gas-Barrier (BGB) is the BM + the CMs of the endothelium respiratory capillaries & the type I cells lining the internal surface of the alveoli. The pulmonary capillaries dilate in areas of high O_2 concentration providing the maximum surface area for gas exchange.

The arterioles bring deoxygenated B to the alveoli;

The capillaries are the site of oxygenation

&

The venules take oxygenated B back to the heart.

1 **terminal bronchiole**
2 **alveolar capillary bed**
3 **pulmonary venule**
4 **alveoli**
5 **pulmonary arteriole**

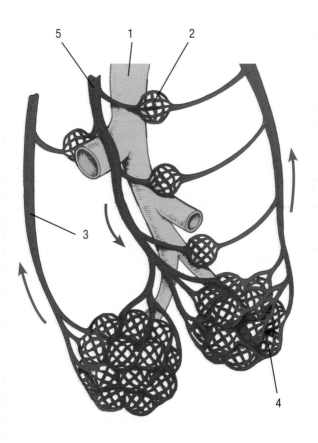

Alveolar Cells - Type I & II in situ

A Diagram of alveolus with type I & II alveolar cells & alveolar capillaries

A Diagram type II alveolar cell showing surfactant production

Type I cells line the inside of the alveolus & Type II cells produce surfactant which coats the Type I cells & the inside of the alveolus reducing its surface tension. Expansion is facilitated. FFAs (free fatty acids), G (glucose), C (choline) & AAs (amino acids) are actively transported from the capillaries to the cell.

1 **capillary endothelium**
2 **capillary lumen**
3 **tight junctional complexes (TJ)**
4 **BM fusion (from the type I & II cells and the endothelium)**
5 **type I alveolar cell**
6 **type II alveolar cell**
7 **macrophage (AKA Type III)**
8 **fibroblast**
9 **large lamellar bodies releasing contents onto the surface**
10 **surfactant - SPs**
11 **alveolar lumen**
12 **GA - releasing small lamellar bodies**
13 **lamellar bodies coalescing**

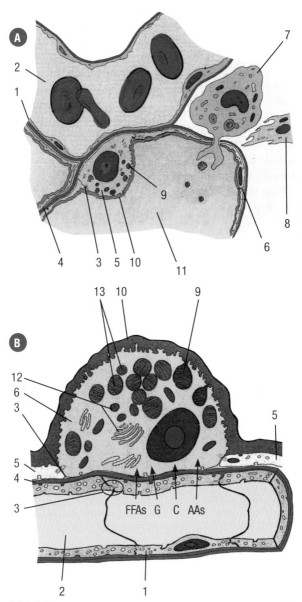

FFAs G C AAs

© A. L. Neill

Alveolus - Gas Exchange (GE)

A Diagram of BS of the alveoli

B Diagram of gas exchange w/n the alveolus via
concentration gradient

O_2 from the atmosphere enters the alveoli, dissolves in the fluid coating the internal surface, and crosses into the capillaries. It is captured in the RBCs via their haemoglobin molecules in exchange for their CO_2

The released CO_2 crosses to the alveoli where it is exhaled. Differences in concentrations drive this process.

1 **bronchiole**
      s = smooth m fibres
2 **venule**
3 **arteriole**
4 **capillary**
5 **alveolar tissue**
6 **RBC**
7 **CO_2**
8 **O_2**
9 **air**

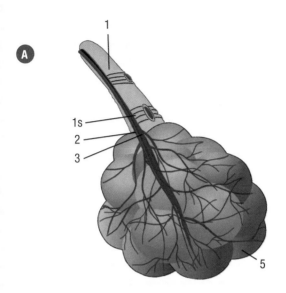

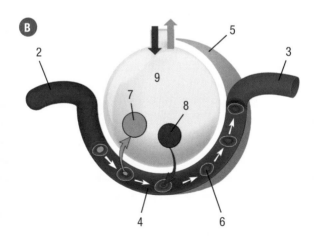

Costovertebral joints AKA Rib/Spine joints of a typical rib

Diagram of joints b/n the ribs & VC superior view

A - the boney joints of rib & VC

B - the ligaments supporting the joints

The typical ribs articulate with the vertebra in 3 places - on the body as demifacets with the VB of their name and the one above - i.e. Rib 3 with the bodies of T2/3 & the TP of the vertebra of the same name, i.e. T3 with Rib 3 .

The BS & NS are segmental from the posterior intercostal arteries, branches of the posterior aorta & posterior intercostal Ns, branches of the spinal Ns (C8-T12)

Due to the changing angles of the joints & the increasing diameter of the ribs the actions of the ribs vary with position

The upper 6 ribs elevate - pump handle action

The lower 4 ribs evert - bucket handle action

The lowest 2 ribs do not move - they anchor the thoracic cage

1 **articular facet for the (TP) transverse process**
2 **tubercle of rib**
3 **articular part of rib**
4 **neck of rib**
5 **facet on the head of the rib**
6 **superior demi-facet on the base of the VB**
7 **articular capsule of the costotransverse jt**
8 **costotransverse lig.**
9 **joint capsule**
10 **intervertebral disc inner - nucleus pulposis**
11 **intervertebral disc outer - annulus fibrosis**
12 **intra-articular lig.**
13 **superior costotransverse lig.**
14 **lat. costotransverse lig.**

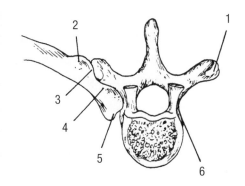

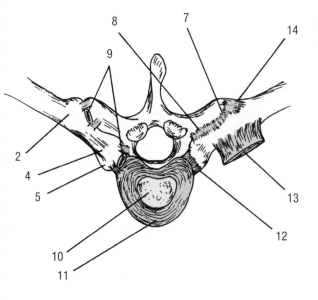

Costovertebral joints AKA Rib/Spine joints of a typical rib

Diagram of joints b/n the ribs & VC lateral view

The typical ribs articulate with the vertebra in 3 places - on the VB as demifacets with the VB of their name and the one above - i.e. Rib 3 with T2/3 & the TP of the vertebra of the same name, i.e. T3 with Rib 3.

Due to the changing angles of the joints & the increasing diameter of the ribs the actions of the ribs vary with position

The upper 6 ribs elevate - pump handle action

The lower 4 ribs evert - bucket handle action

The lowest 2 ribs do not move

A - the boney joints of rib & VC

B - the ligaments supporting the joints

1   **articular facet for TP**
2   **superior demi-facet on the base of the VB**
3   **VB = vertebral body**
4   **radiate lig.**
5   **ALL = anterior longitudinal lig.**
6   **intervertebral disc**
7   **intra-articular lig.**
8   **head of rib**
9   **angle and shaft of rib**
10   **paired synovial joints planar with demi-facets**
11   **superior costotransverse lig.**
12   **spine of thoracic vertebra**
13   **superior costo-demi-facet on inferior aspect of VB**

See CT for further clarification

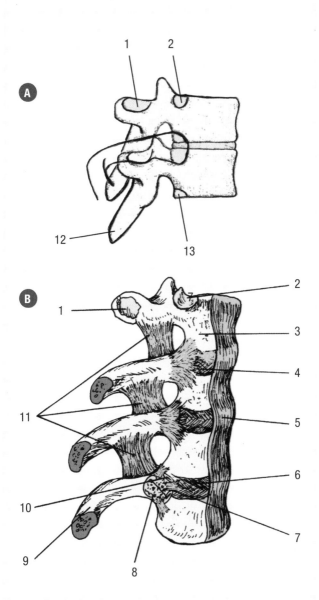

Rib (5) - articulations

Diagram of joints of the 5th rib - a Typical rib

Rib 5 articulates with the VC at the levels of T4/5 & the Sternum via the costal cartilage.

1 **jugular notch - of the Manubrium**
2 **articular demifacets for rib 2**
3 **manubriosternal jt AKA Sternal angle**
4 **Sternum**
5 **Rib 5**
6 **body of T6 ie VB of T6**
7 **costal cartilage of rib 5**
8 **Xiphoid process**
9 **demifacets for rib articulation i = inferior / s = superior**
10 **facet on the TP of T4 for rib 4**
11 **SP of T4 - note points downwards**
12 **Xiphoid process**
13 **xiphisternal jts**

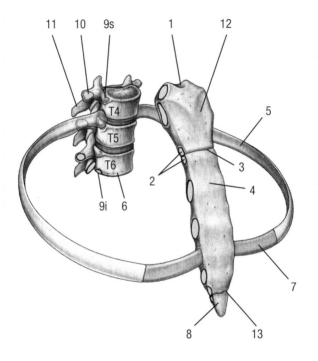

Ribs 1-2 - atypical features

A - articulations - superior view

B - separated bones - superior view

Ribs 1,2 are atypical ribs.

Rib 1 does not move with respiration & only articulates with T1, it is a small stout rib

Rib 2 is larger & articulates at the sternal angle

1/1A	**T1 - RIB 1**
2/2A	**T2 RIB 2**
3	**costovertebral joints**
3A	**demi-facets on head of Rib 2 b/n T1 and T2 crest in b/n**
	single facet on head of Rib 1 for T1
4	**spine of T1 + TP**
5	**costal tubercles**
6	**shafts**
7A /7V	**groove for subclavian artery and N and vein**
8	**scalene tubercle**
9	**attachment of costovertebral lig.**
10	**attachment of lig. of Serratus Anterior**

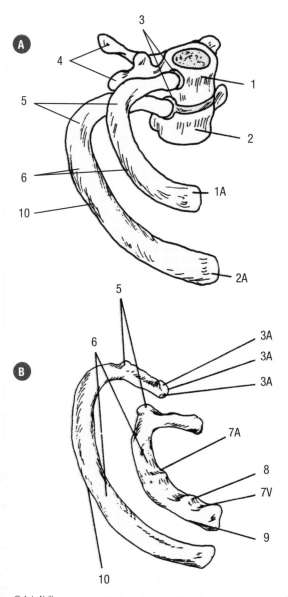

Rib - typical features

A - Anterior view cartilage attached

B - Inferior view

C - Posterior view

Ribs 3-10 are typical ribs. They articulate with the VC in 3 places and with the manubriosternum via the costal cartilage.

1 **head**
2 **neck**
3 **tubercle facet**
4 **tubercle**
5 **angle of the rib**
6 **shaft / body of rib**
7 **costal groove**
8 **costal end**
9 **inferior demi- facet**
10 **interarticular crest**
11 **superior demi-facet**
12 **costal cartilage**

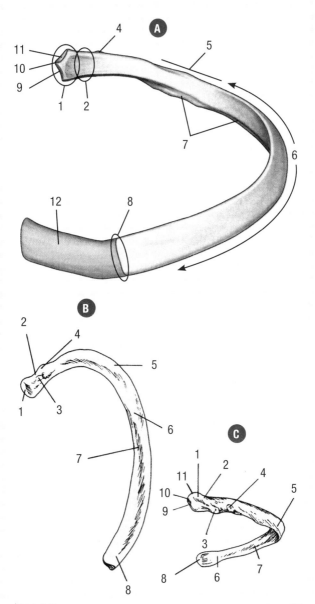

Manubriosternum = Manubrium + Sternum + Xiphoid process AKA Breast bone

Anterior & lateral view of the Breast bone

1 **Manubrium b**
2 **clavicular notch**
3 **notch for 1st CC (rib)**
4 **notch for 2nd rib**
5 **sternal angle / manubriosternal jt - angle of Louis**
6 **notch for 3rd CC**
7 **notch for 4th CC**
8 **notch for 5th CC**
9 **notch for 6th CC**
10 **notch for 7th CC**
11 **Xiphoid process**
12 **xiphisternal jt**
13 **Sternum b**
14 **jugular notch**

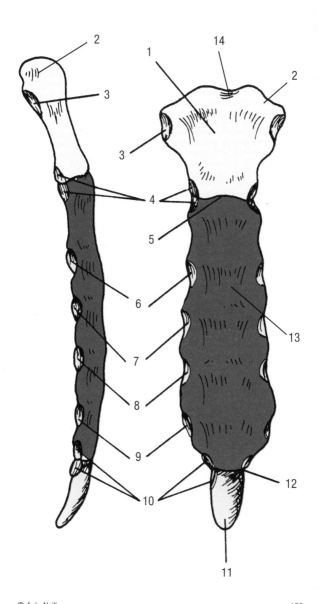

Manubriosternum joints

A - Anterior view of the manubrio-costal & manubrio-clavicular joints

B - Anterior view of the sterno-costal joints

The Sternum articulates with the ribs & allows for elevation/ depression, retraction/ protraction & rotation. All movements are needed in respiration - & the shoulder movements involving the Clavicle

1 interclavicular lig
2 articular surface
3 intra-articular disc- cartilagenous disc w/n the jt
4 costo-clavicular lig
5 double synovial jt cavity RIB 2 with intra-articular lig, manubrio-costal / sterno-costal jts
6 manubriosternal symphysis (20 cartilaginous)
7 ant. sternoclavicular lig
8 radiate costo-clavicular lig
9 radiate sterno-costal lig
10 sterno-costal joints (R3-9) PLANE synovial joints
11 interchondral synovial joint cavities (R6-10) synchondrosis
12 interchondral ligs syndesmosis
13 costo-chondral junction

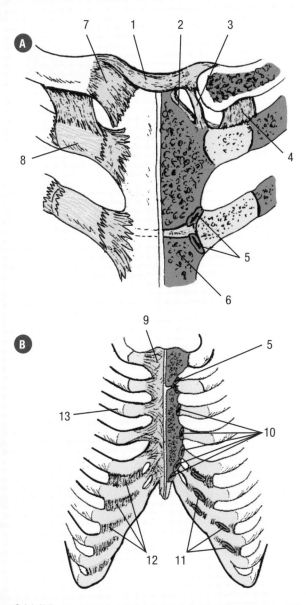

Thoracic Spine - Ligaments of

A - Posterior view of the thoracic spine - looking at the back - skin & superficial T removed

B - Superior view of the thoracic vertebra (upper region)

C - Transverse section through the thoracic vertebra (lower region)

The thoracic spine is the most protected region of the SC, via its ligs & down-pointing SPs, protecting the delicate lung T underneath. It transforms from cervical-like vertebrae to lumbar-like vertebrae as the SPs become smaller, straighter & thicker. It is also relatively immobile, due mainly to the costo-vertebral joints.

1 supra-spinous lig.(supf to the inter-spinous lig.)
2 TP
3 lat. costo-transverse lig.
4 superior costo-transverse lig.
5 capsular lig. of zygapophyseal jt
6 inter-laminar ligs - deep & supf - maybe split
7 part of the radiate lig - covers the demifacets of the costo-vertebral jts
8 supf. costo-vertebral lig.
9 inter-transverse process lig.
10 lamina
11 rib
12 articular pillar
13 costo-vertebral lig. AKA radiate lig. covering vertebral demifacets
14 costo-transverse lig.
15 artic. facet of zygapophyseal jt
16 costo-vertebral jt - demi-facet on VB
17 lateral costo-vertebral jt
18 SP
19 body of the thoracic vertebra
20 vertebral canal
21 ligamentum flavum AKA yellow lig.
22 PLL
23 ALL

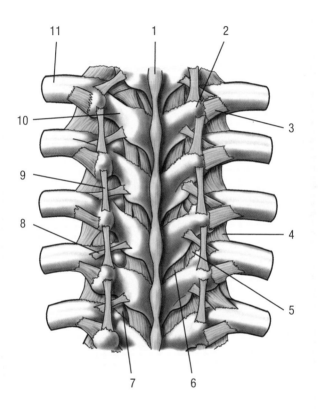

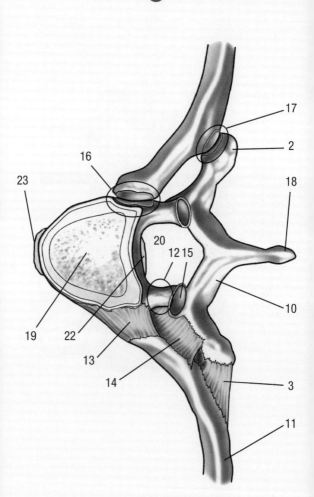

© A. L. Neill

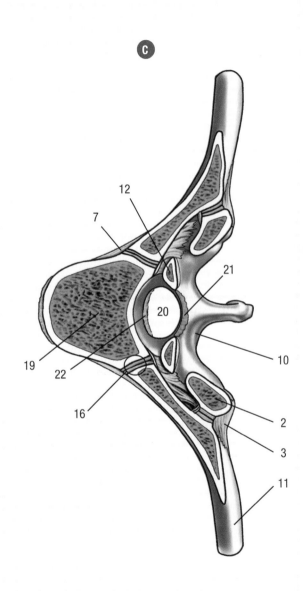

Bronchial Tree

Macroscopic view of the conducting passages

A - Larynx

B - Trachea

C - Bronchial tree

Before there can be any GE the air must be transported to the alveoli via the conducting passages. These passages branch to form smaller & smaller segments called "generation" of which there are b/n 16-20. They maintain their cartilage until bronchioles at the end of the TZ & the beginning of the RZ. There are 3 lobes on the R side reflected by the 3 lobar bronchi & only 2 on L due to the heart.

1 **Hyoid**

2 **thyroid cartligae**

3 **cricoid cartilage**

4 **tracheal cartilage**

5 **annular intercartilage lig**

6 **main bronchus**

    L = left - more horizontal due to the heart

    R = right - straighter - more likely for food or particles to enter from this side

7 **L superior lobar bronchus**

8 **L superior segmental bronchus**

9 **L inferior lobar bronchus**

10 **tracheal carina = tracheal bifurcation**

11 **R segmental bronchus - this is the smallest anatomical unit of the lung**

12 **R middle lobar bronchus**

13 **median cricothyroid ligament**

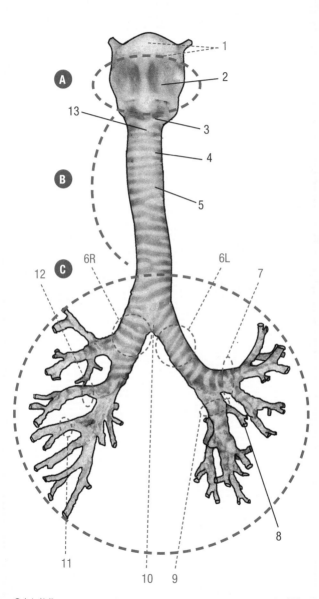

Divisions of the Bronchial tree

X + T = total lung capacity (TLC)

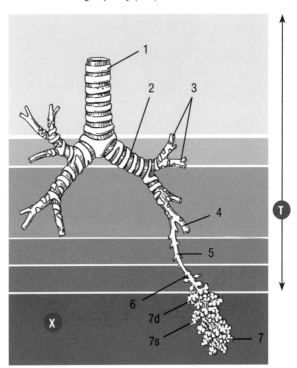

T = transport zone (TZ)   X = respiratory zone (RZ) region of GE

1 **trachea**
2 **10 bronchi**
3 **lobar bronchi**
4 **segmental bronchi**
5 **terminal bronchiole**
6 **respiratory bronchiole**
7 **alveolus**
d = duct / s = sac

RZ = from terminal bronchioles to the alveoli, each forming a TRU AKA acinus, the smallest individual respiratory unit.

© A. L. Neill

Histological features

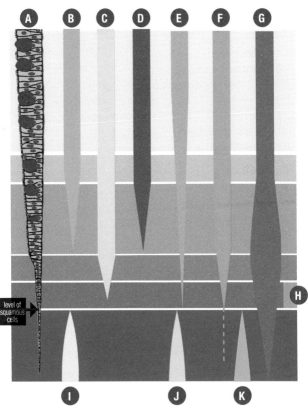

A - epithelium
B - goblet cells B/A = 1/5 =
    Reid index*
C - ciliated cells + brush
    cells
D - glands (mixed)
E - cartilage

F - smooth muscle
G - elastic fibres
H - Clara cells / canals of
    Lambert
I - type I cells
J - type II cells
K - type III cells

Reid Index = 1 : 5 - goblet cells to epithelial cells, this increases in asthma &
bronchitis

© A. L. Neill

Respiratory passages

A - intrapulmonary bronchus MP - H&E

B - terminal bronchiole (end of TZ) HP - H&E

Air is transported from the outside to the alveoli via a series of passages which become smaller & smaller, reducing their wall structure progressively through the respiratory tree: commencing with the trachea → bronchi → bronchioles → alveolar sacs. B/n the bronchi & the bronchioles cartilage is lost in the wall & the lining cells change from pseudostratified columnar epithelial cell to simple columnar cells.*

1   **alveoli**
2   **hyaline cartilage + epichondrium**
3   **pulmonary v**
4   **submucosal glands**
5   **mucosa**
6   **adipose T**
7   **PSCCE**
8   **pulmonary a**
9   **serous glands + ducts**
10 **muscularis - smooth m**
11 **columnar epithelium - quickly flattens in the RZ**
12 **lamina propria - of the mucosa + submucosa**

* Each terminal bronchiole opens to 10,000 alveoli and forms a single acinus (TRU)

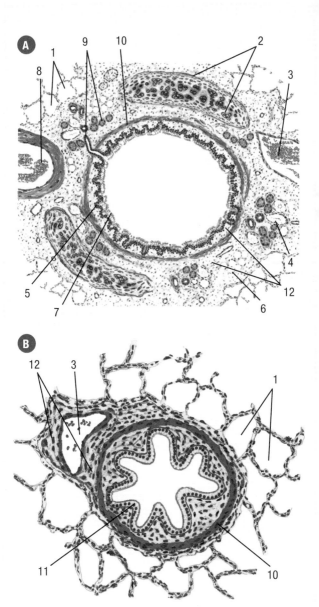

Bronchioles (TRU)

Normal

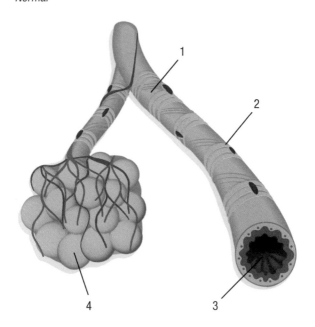

In the asthmatic / atopic patient the bronchioles (1) tighten (smooth muscle contraction - 2), the MM swells (3t) & ↑ secretions (3m), reducing the airflow, & increasing the effort to breathe. The alveoli (4) are not filled ↓↓ GE (4s).

1 **bronchiole**
2 **smooth muscle t = contracting**
3 **mucus membrane t = swollen / m = mucus secretion**
4 **alveoli s = smaller / under ventilated**

Bronchioles (TRU)

Inflamed (Asthmatic)

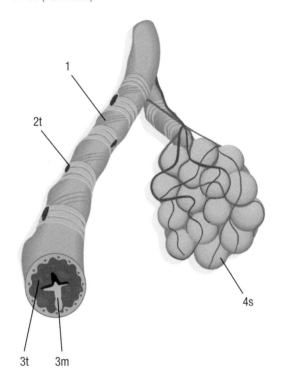

1

2t

3t   3m

4s

Terminal Bronchiole - Elastic fibres & Smooth Muscle

Diagram of terminal bronchiole & alveoli showing elastic fibre & smooth muscle cell relationships

The elastic fibres allow for the large volume changes of the lungs. They are found throughout the lung T arranged longitudinally around the bronchioles & in a network through the alveoli. The smooth muscle cells are arranged helically around the bronchioles and only intermittant in most alveoli.

A - Pulmonary lobule

B - Pulmonary acinus

1 **terminal bronchiole**

2 **smooth muscle cells - concentric**

3 **elastic fibres - longitudinal**

4 **respiratory bronchiole with alveolar buds 4a and canals of Lambert 4c connecting bronchiole & alveoli**

5 **alveolar duct - containing 50% of all alveoli 16-20 for each duct**

6 **alveolar sac**

7 **alveolus L = lumen - with 65% of all GE due to its increased SA**

8 **alveolar pores AKA Pores of Kohn, connect adjacent alveoli, responsible for collateral respiration in case of blockage**

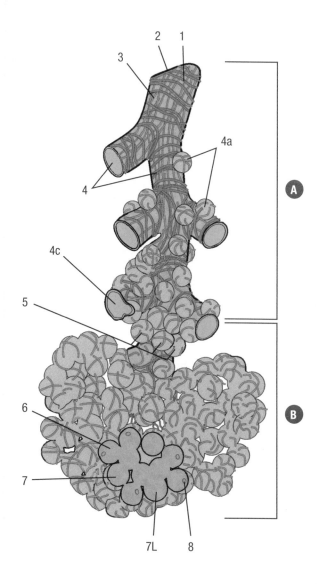

Terminal Lobule - Structure

Diagram of terminal lobule & the visceral pleura (adherant pleural layer)

The terminal lobule has its own BS & NS and is closely related to the visceral pleura. The expanding rib cage pulls on this pleura & expands the lung T.

1 **terminal bronchiole**
2 **respiratory bronchiole**
3 **alveolar duct**
4 **alveolus**
5 **capillary bed**
6 **alveolar pores AKA Pores of Kohn, connect adjacent alveoli**
7 **elastic fibres**
8 **visceral pleura**
9 **smooth muscle - peribronchiolar fascia supporting up to 10,000 alveoli**
10 **bronchiolar lymphatic**
11 **bronchiolar v**
12 **bronchiolar a**
13 **canal of Lambert**
14 **common septa pf alveoli**
15 **alveolar cornices with Type II cells**

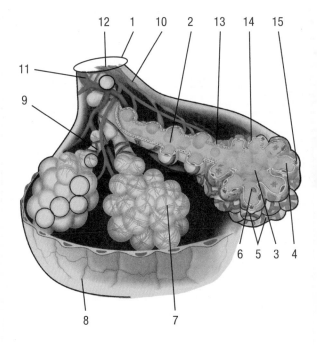

Bronchopulmonary segments & lobes - anterior & posterior

The bronchopulmonary segment is the smallest functioning unit in the lung capable of being removed in surgery. Some variation exists in these segments although not with the lobes - please note posterior view is flipped over.

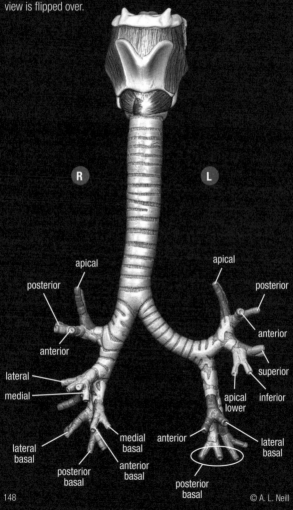

R

L

apical

apical

posterior

posterior

anterior

anterior

superior

inferior

lateral

apical lower

medial

lateral basal

medial basal

anterior

lateral basal

posterior basal

anterior basal

posterior basal

148

© A. L. Neill

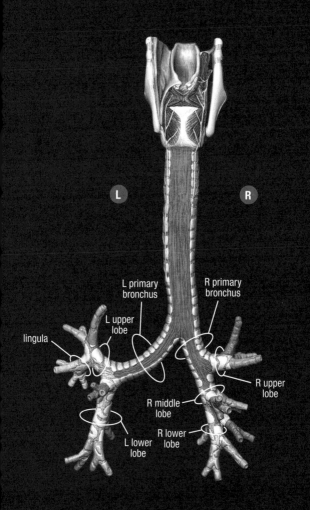

L primary bronchus

R primary bronchus

L upper lobe

lingula

R upper lobe

R middle lobe

R lower lobe

L lower lobe

© A. L. Neill

Bronchus

Diagram of a bronchus with the adventitia removed to show the cartilage plates

The bronchus differs from the trachea, in its cartilaginous plates, smaller lumen, orientation of its smooth muscle and increased amounts of elastic T. The smooth muscle extends to the alveoli along with the elastic fibres, & wraps around the lumen. Muscle contraction causes the mucosa to fold longitudinally in this region.

1 **hyaline cartilage plates**
2 **mucous & serous glands**
3 **CT containing lymphoid T**
4 **smooth muscle - helical**
5 **elastic fibres in areolar T - longitudinal**
6 **bronchial lumen**
7 **mucosal longitudinal folds - columnar epithelium**
8 **lumen of bronchlole - mucus from here is sputum and swept up to the carina by ciliated cells**

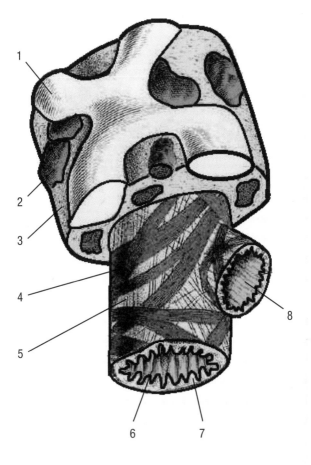

Carina

Diagram of carina in situ - & superior view

The carina is the site of the primary bronchi formation - the bifurcation of the trachea. The ciliated epithelium sweep sputum or phlegm towards this area; the site of the coughing reflex(10).

The glottis closes building up the pressure & then opens to spurt/cough the mucous out of the RT. Similar events occur in the gag reflex.

1   **oesophagus**
2   **L recurrent laryngeal N**
3   **trachea**
4   **L subclavian a**
5   **L Vagus N**
6   **arch of the aorta (oxygenated B going to the body)**
7   **ligamentum arteriosus (remnants of the intrauterine pulmonary bypass)**
8   **main bronchus (L&R)**
9   **pulmonary trunk (deoxygenated B going to the lungs) recurrent laryngeal N**
10 **carina**

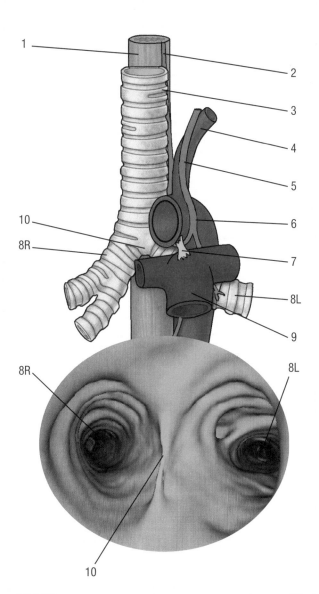

Head & Neck cavities

Relationship in the head & its cavities

This is a section of the head - with the anterior quarter removed to show the relationship b/n the muscles & cavities.*

1   **olfactory bulb - & N (CN I)**
2   **N processes in the nasal cavity**
3   **conchae (turbinates) superior, middle & inferior**
4   **nostril region - limit of the digital penetration**
5   **hard palate**
6   **oral cavity**
7   **tongue**
8   **epiglottis**
9   **tracheal cartilages**
10 **oesophagus**
11 **larynx**
12 **pharynx**
13 **oropharynx**
14 **uvula**
15 **soft palate**
16 **Eustachian tube**
17 **pituitary gland**
18 **brain**

* Note the frontal and ethmoid sinuses.

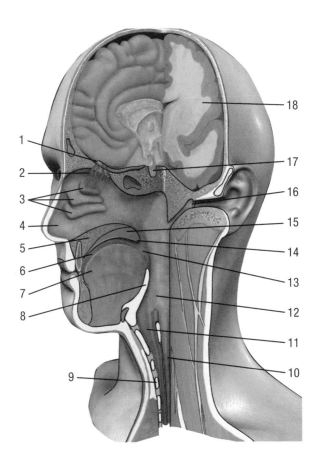

1 —

2 —

3 —

4 —

5 —

6 —

7 —

8 —

9 —

— 18

— 17

— 16

— 15

— 14

— 13

— 12

— 11

— 10

Epiglottis

Sagittal view - looking onto a cut section of the epiglottis showing the lingual and laryngeal surfaces LP

HP sections of the epiglottis :

A - taste bud on the lingual surface surrounded by stratified squamous epithelium

B - stratified squamous epithelium on the laryngeal surface

C - pseudo-stratified ciliated columnar epithelium (PSCCE)

The larynx is lined by epithelial cells which undergo changes when stressed. The taste buds present on the surface are thought to act as stimulation of the gag reflex.

1 **mucosa - containing fat cells & mixed glands**
2 **perichondrium**
3 **fibro cartilage - containing high amounts of elastic fibres**
4 **lamina propria**
5 **lymph nodules**
6 **mucous glands**

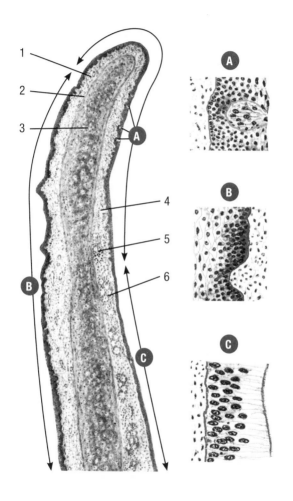

Hyoid bone & Larynx

Anterolateral view - looked at from the front & side

The thyroid cartilage is the most prominent feature of the neck - Adam's apple. ♀ < ♂

The Hyoid is the only bone which does not articulate with another bone.

1 **Hyoid b**
2 **cricoid cart. - only complete cartilagenous ring**
3 **thyroid cart.**
4 **thyro-hyoid mem.**
5 **crico-tracheal lig.**
6 **hypoepiglottic lig.**
7 **epiglottis**
8 **tracheal cartilage (incomplete ring)**
9 **lesser horn (cornu)**
10 **greater horn (cornu)**

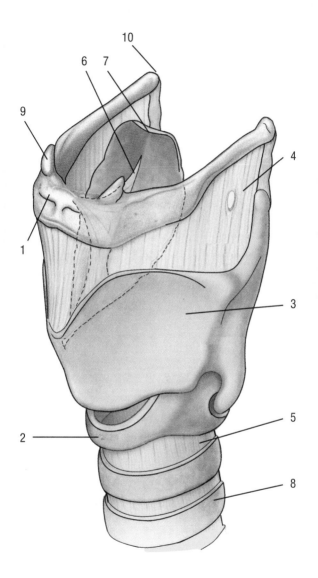

Larynx - in situ

A - Anterolateral view - looking onto larynx from the front & side superficial structures removed

B - Anterior view of the surface anatomy of the larynx & trachea

C - Lateral view of surface anatomy of larynx & trachea - female/male

The Hyoid, superior thyroid notch laryngeal prominence AKA Adam's apple are palpable in the neck. B/n the thyroid & cricoid cartilages is the crico-thyroid membrane; the site of access to the trachea inferior to the larynx*. The oesophagus is intimately associated with the posterior of the trachea, which along with the great vessels descends into the thorax through the superior thoracic outlet.

1 **stylohyoid lig**

2 **Hyoid b**

3 **pharyngeal constrictors m**
    i = inferior
    m = middle
    s = superior

4 **oesophagus**

5 **trachea**

6 **crico thyroid m / overlying cricoid cart**

7 **crico-thyroid membrane AKA crico-vocal membrane**

8 **laryngeal prominence & notch**

9 **laryngeal cart. AKA thyroid cart.**

10 **thyro-hyoid membrane**

11 **epiglottis**

12 **first cartilage of the trachea - incomplete cartilage ring, posterior wall related to anterior wall of the oesophagus**

13 **thyroid gland which consists of 2 lobes connected by the**
    i = isthmus passing across the trachea

14 **medial border of the SCM m**

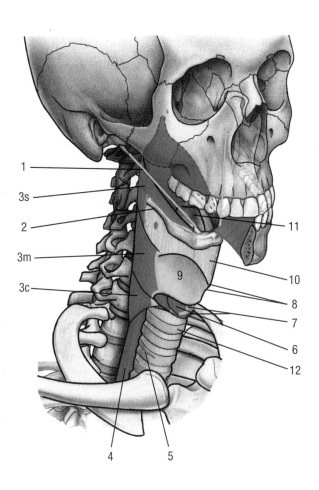

B

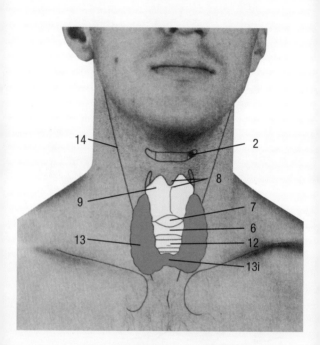

© A. L. Neill

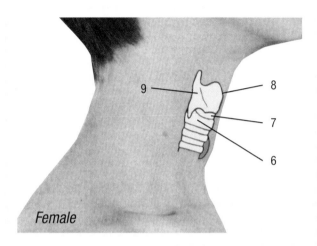

9
8
7
6

Female

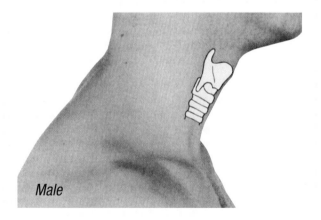

Male

Larynx - Trachea relationship

Posterior view - looking onto the anterior larynx - coronal section - muscles & surrounding CT removed - diagram

The larynx is superior to the trachea and hence if closed will prevent breathing. Inferior to the thyroid cartilage is the crico-thyroid ligament, a site suitable for opening to allow air into the trachea with a closed larynx.

Areas which are irritated change their ciliated columnar mucosal surface for a more resilient stratified squamous epithelium, which is dryer & does not have the capacity to clear the airway of dust. This may result in a persistent dry cough, causing more trauma.

1 **epiglottis**

    c = simple columnar epithelial surface

    s = stratified squamous epithelial surface

2 **vestibule AKA anterior commissure**

3 **thyroid cart. AKA laryngeal cart.**

4 **laryngeal saccule**

5 **laryngeal ventricle**

6 **Reinke's space - site of vocalis muscle (m)**

7 **crico-thyroid membrane AKA crico-vocal membrane**

8 **infraglottic space**

9 **site of tracheotomy**

10 **vestibular fold AKA false vocal cord**

    s = stratified squamous epithelial surface

11 **vocal fold AKA true vocal cord**

    s = stratified epithelial surface if strained from irritants or over use - columnar epithelium when rested or non traumatized - reduced use

12 **trachea - surface of ciliated columnar epithelium (c) - changes to a squamous epithelium when irritated eg smokers with increased mucosal secretions**

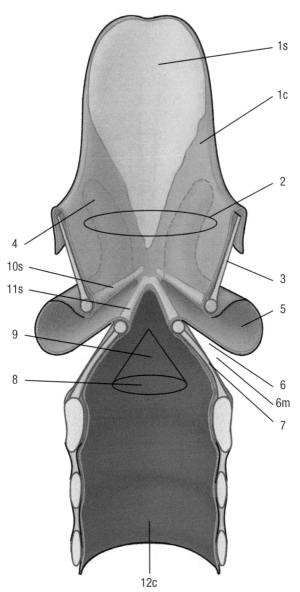

Larynx Cartilage and Fascia

Superior view - looked at from above

The VCs are more medial than the other ligs of this structure. Air passing through these cords results in voice.

The epiglottis closes off the trachea when food or liquid is being swallowed.

1 **thyroid cart.**
2 **epiglottis**
3 **arytenoid cart.**
4 **corniculate cart.**
5 **cuneiform cart.**
6 **crico-thyroid lig. AKA cricovocal lig.**
7 **chorda vocalis AKA vocal cord - free edge of the lig. AKA vocal lig.**
8 **quadrangular membrane**
9 **cricoid cart.**
10 **vestibular lig.**

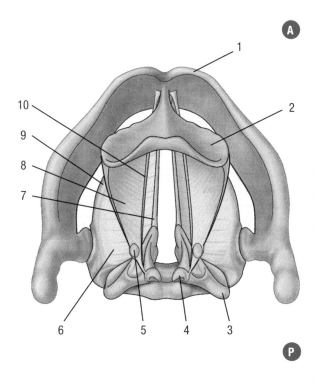

Larynx - cartilages & muscle

Interior - Superior view - looked at from above

When the laryngeal muscles are relaxed the rima glottidis is closed & the person cannot breathe.

1 cricoid cartilage
2 superior cornu (horn) of the thyroid cart.
3 arytenoid cart.
4 upper margin of thyroid cart.
5 body of thyroid cart.
6 cricoid cart.
7 chorda vocalis AKA vocal cord (R&L)
8 Thyro-arytenoideus m
9 Crico-arytenoideus lateralis m
10 Crico-arytenoideus posterior m (R & L)
11 rima glottidis AKA structures surrounding glottis
12 Arytenoideus m

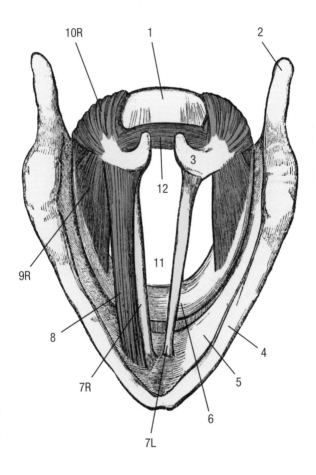

Larynx - Blood Supply

Arterial supply

Lateral view with cartilage wall removed to show inside
Medial view - cartilage wall removed

The BS of the larynx, parathyroid and thyroid are related intimately. Hence voice changes may be a sign of pathologies in these areas.

1   **carotid arteries c = common / e = external /
    i = internal**
2   **lingual arteries**
3   **hyoid arteries i = infrahyoid / s = suprahyoid art**
4   **laryngeal i = inferior / s = superior**
5   **thyroid art i = inferior / s = superior**
6   **cricothyroid m**
7   **thyrocervical trunk**
8   **subclavian**
9   **aorta**
10 **Hyoid**
11 **cricoid cart**
12 **epiglottis**
13 **thyroid**
14 **trachea**

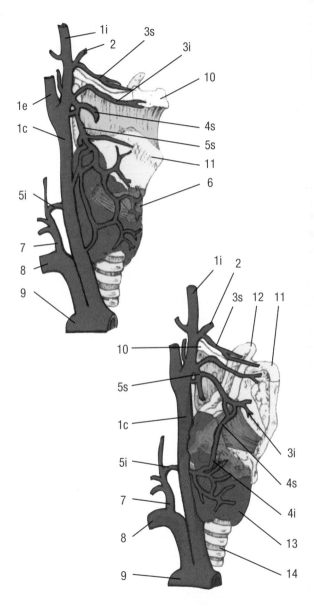

Larynx - Nerve supply

A = *anterior*

B = *posterior*

C = *superior*

1 **Hyoid b**
2 **thyroid cart.**
3 **R Vagus N**
4 **R recurrent laryngeal N**
5 **L recurrent laryngeal N**
6 **L Vagus N**
7 **VCs**
8 **posterior branch of inf. laryngeal N**
9 **anterior branch of inf. laryngeal N**
10 **posterior muscle band of trachea**
11 **superior laryngeal N**
12 **internal branch of superior laryngeal N**
13 **external branch of superior laryngeal N**

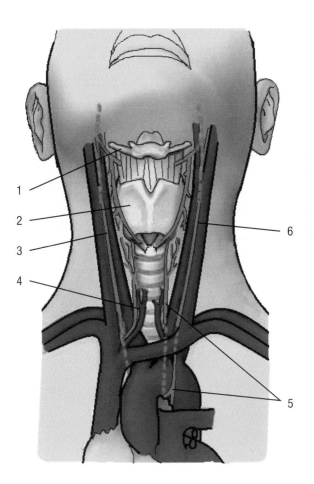

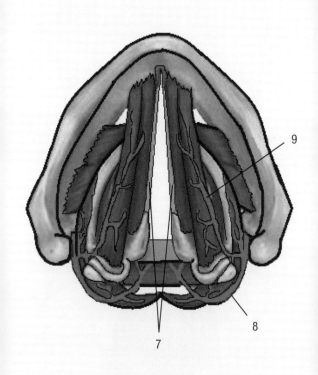

9

8

7

B

© A. L. Neill

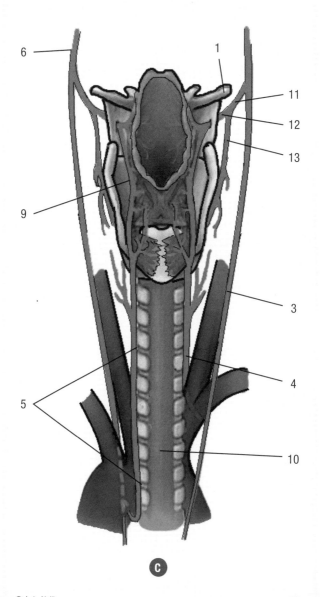

C

© A. L. Neill

Larynx - microanatomy

Sagittal view - looking onto the larynx from the side

The larynx is lined by epithelial cells which undergo changes when stressed.

1　adipose T
2　BVs arteriole & venule
3　lamina propria of the ventricle
4　serous glands
5　mucous glands
4 + 5　mixed glands
6　lymph nodules AKA laryngeal tonsils
7　thyroid cart. AKA laryngeal cart.
　　　　p = perichondrium
8　thyroarytenoid m (skeletal muscle)
9　cricoid cart.
10　vocal folds f　= false cords t = true cords
11　vestibule AKA space b/n the vocal folds
12　epiglottis - post. surface
13　junction b/n pseudo-columnar ciliated epithelial lining of the larynx & stratified squamous epithelium
14　vocalis m

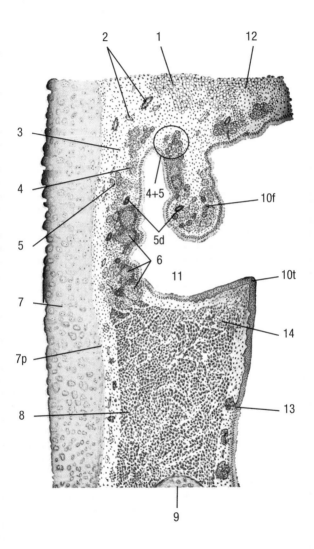

Lungs - displayed

Anterior view - with lungs displaced to show relationship with heart & great vessels

The lungs are intimately related to the heart & great vessels - the origins of which are shown here. Retracting the lungs exposes the anterior heart surface. With the pericardium removed the chambers of the heart can be identified & related to the origins of the vessels

1. first rib (L&R)
2. subclavian a&v (L&R)
3. L lung - d =lower lobe / u = upper lobe
4. phrenic neurovascular bundle - (a&v&N)
5. pleural space
   (space b/n the 2 pleural layers -containing the lungs)
6. diaphragm c = central tendon / m = muscular domes
7. R lung - d =lower lobe / m = middle lobe / u = upper lobe
8. SVC
9. aorta
10. pulmonary arterial trunk
    b/n 8,9 & 10 lies the thymus
11. ligamentum arteriosum - remnant of foetal pulmonary bypass
12. parietal pleura (adherent to the thoracic wall) - note it lies above the first rib
13. brachial plexus
    14 + 15 + 16 + 17 = chambers of the heart
14. RA
15. RV
16. LV
17. LA

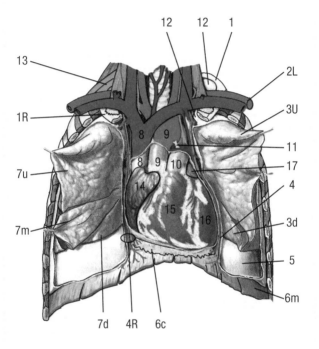

Lungs

A - Anterior view - lungs in situ surface structures removed
B - Medial view looking onto the root of the R lung
C - Medial view looking onto the root of the L lung

The lungs occupy most of the thoracic cavity. The pleural sacs wrap the lung parenchymal tissue & then coat the inner surface of the ribs & IC muscles, as a double sac. It is the negative pressure generated by the rib cage expansion that draws air in. The lungs are the site of blood oxygenation. Organs & BVs passing through the thorax leave impressions on the surface of these soft pliable organs.

1 **cricoid cart.**
2 **thyroid gld**
3 **L lung**
    i = superior lobe
    ii = cardiac notch
    iii = inferior lobe
4 **IC muscles**
5 **parietal pleural lining**
6 **oblique fissure b/n the 2 lobes**
7 **pericardium**
8 **thymus**
9 **diaphragm r = recess**
10 **R lung**
    i = superior lobe
    ii = middle lobe
    iii = inferior lobe
11 **first rib**
12 **trachea**
13 **root of the lung**
14 **pulmonary v**
15 **pulmonary a**
16 **main bronchus**
17 **hilar LNs AKA broncho-pulmonary LNs**

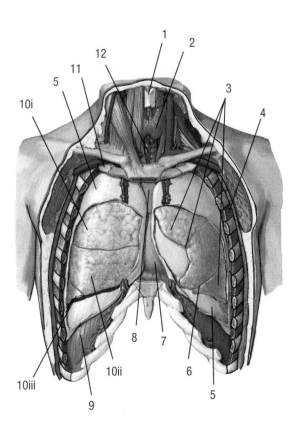

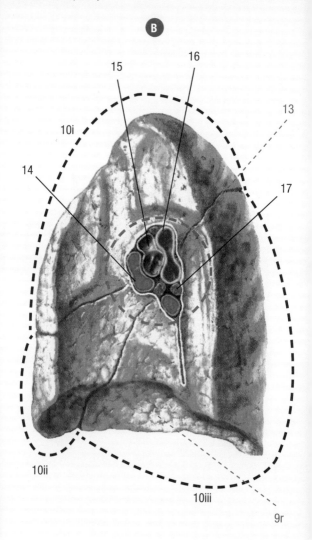

© A. L. Neill

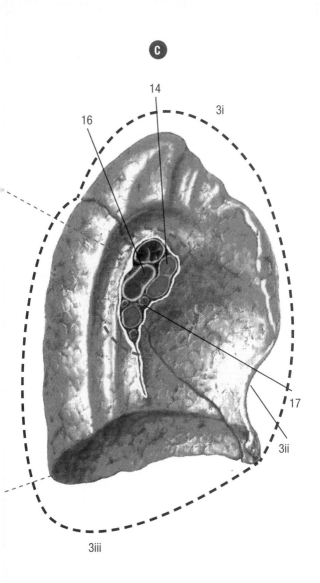

C

14

16

3i

17

3ii

3iii

Lungs - in situ

Transverse section of thoracic cavity at the level of T6

The lungs sit in the thorax on either side of the heart. A framework of muscles surrounds the cavity & supplies the UL shoulders & back

1   **heart**
2   **lungs R & L**
3   **oesophagus**
4   **aorta (descending)**
5   **trachea**
6   **T6**
7   **SC**
8   **pleural lining**
9   **pericardium**

© A. L. Neill

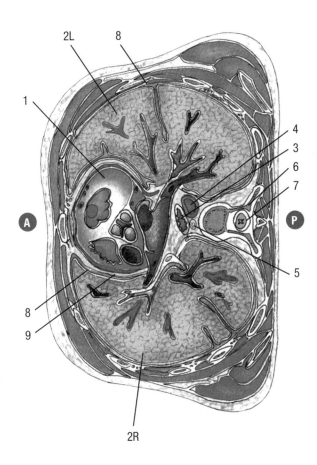

2L

8

1

4

3

6

7

A

P

8

9

5

2R

© A. L. Neill

Lung parenchyma

*Transverse section LP H&E of the lung tissue showing –
alveolar tissue, bronchioles & most of the structures of the
lower respiratory tract*

The lung is a soft aerated T composed of small thin walled sacs - the
alveoli. It is here that the gases are exchanged along concentration
lines - via slow flowing ↓ P capillaries.

1   **serosa = visceral pleura**
     c = inner layer of CT & BVs
     m = outer layer mesothelium
2   **alveolar duct**
3   **respiratory bronchiole**
4   **alveolus - area of gas exchange**
5   **terminal bronchiole + pulmonary vein**
6   **pulmonary a & v**
7   **bronchial hyaline cartilage plates**
8   **bronchial glands with ducts**
9   **bronchus - lumen**
10 **pseudostratified epithelial lining with underlying mucosa**
11 **smooth m**
12 **submucosa**
13 **adventitia**
14 **lymphatic nodule**
15 **mucosal folds**
16 **trabeculae + BVs**
17 **alveolar sacs**

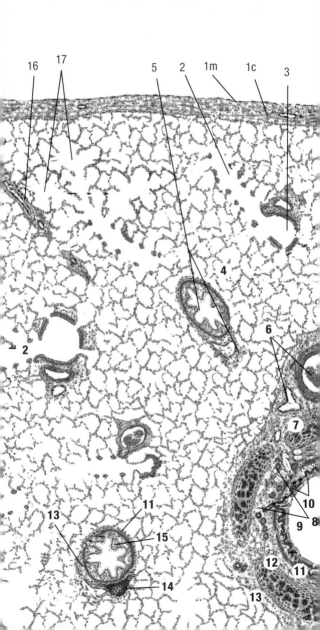

Lungs & Pleura - Surface Anatomy

Anterior view of the chest showing lung and pleural sac markings

The lungs come above the ribs anteriorly and there is a greater disparity b/n pleura and lungs in the ant. than post.

3 lobes on the R lung – additional fissure

2 lobes on the L lung – cardiac notch

1 **Manubrium – has jts with rib 1 & Clavicle**

2 **outline of lungs**

3 **outline of parietal pleura**

4 **oblique fissure – lungs + visceral pleural makings**

5 **Sternum (1 + 5 = manubriosternum) anchors ribs 2-6 individually & the CC of ribs 7-10**

6 **6th rib**

7 **ribs 7-10 attached via CC to the Sternum**

8 **horizontal fissure – R side 4th ICS**

9 **cardiac notch – L side 4th ICS**

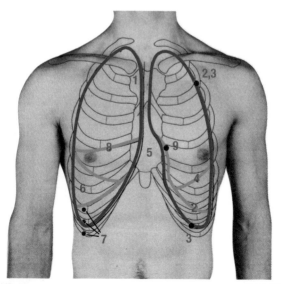

© A. L. Neill

Lungs & Pleura - Surface Anatomy

Posterior view of the chest showing lung and pleural sac markings

The lungs do not come above the ribs posteriorly

3 lobes on the R lung – additional fissure

2 lobes on the L lung – cardiac notch

1 SP of T1 – attached to rib 1
2 outline of lungs
3 outline of parietal pleura
4 oblique fissure – lungs + visceral pleural makings
5 thoracoabdominal incision post.
6 6th rib
7 vertebra prominens – defn – most prominent
    SP (usually C7 rarely C6)
8 distance b/n SPs & lung pleura 2 fingers (2 ½ cm)
9 floating ribs 11,12

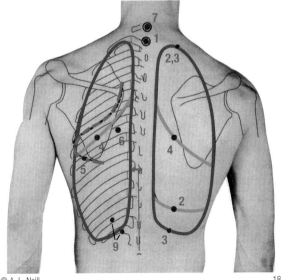

Lymph nodes - of the lungs & bronchi

A diagram of the LNs of the respiratory system, & their pattern of drainage

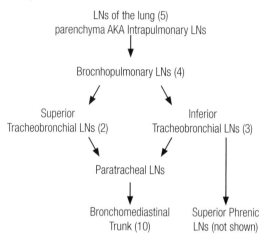

LNs of the lung (5)
parenchyma AKA Intrapulmonary LNs

Brocnhopulmonary LNs (4)

Superior
Tracheobronchial LNs (2)

Inferior
Tracheobronchial LNs (3)

Paratracheal LNs

Bronchomediastinal
Trunk (10)

Superior Phrenic
LNs (not shown)

1 **paratracheal LNs**

2 **superior tracheobronchial LNs**

3 **inferior tracheobronchial LNs AKA interbronchial LNs**

4 **bronchopulmonary LNs -**
   LNs may drain to the opposite side of the chest
   LNs often involved in cancers associated
   with smoking

5 **intrapulmonary LNs**

6 **anterior basal segmental bronchus**

7 **L inf. lobar bronchus**

8 **main bronchus (L&R) R straighter than the L**

9 **trachea**

10 **path leading to the bronchomediastinal trunks (L&R)**

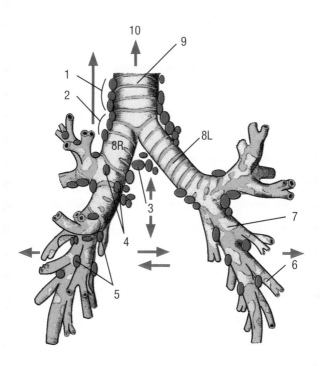

Lung Capacities & Volumes

Internationally agreed names are used to describe volumes that make up breathing & other respiratory measures. Lung Volumes (LVs)

Lung Capacities (LCs) are the sum of 2 or more LVs

Lung Capacities (LCs) :		
INSPIRATORY CAPACITY (IC)	>3,600mls	
TOTAL LUNG CAPACITY (TLC)	>6,000mls	TV + IRV + ERV + RV
VITAL CAPACITY (VC)	>4,800mls	~80% of TLC TV + IRV + ERV
	the max. inspiration + the max. expiration	
FUNCTIONAL RESIDUAL CAPACITY (FRC)	>2,400mls	RV + ERV
	the amount of air left after expiration	

Lung Volumes (LVs) :		
EXPIRARTORY RESERVE VOLUME (ERV)	= 1,200mls	
	additional air that can be exhaled below TV	
INSPRIRATORY RESERVE VOLUME (IRV)	= 3,100mls	
	additional air that can be inhaled above TV	
RESIDUAL VOLUME (RV)	= 1,200mls	volume left after ERV
TIDAL VOLUME(TV)	= 500mls	the average breath volume

Mediastinum Diagrams

A - anterior (looking at)
B - lateral (looking into)
C - superior (looking on top of)

Definition - the thoracic space b/n the lungs

It is further subdivided into 4 components

1 superior – above the heart to the root of the neck

2 anterior – in front of the heart

3 middle – the cavity for the heart

4 posterior – the space behind the heart until the diaphragm (inf. border)

5 **mediastinum = 1 + 2 + 3 + 4**

6 **apex of the lung (above rib 1 & the mediastinum)**

7 **L & R lung**

8 **roots of the lung L& R (pleura folds back on itself - pulmonary trunks pass through)**

9 **pleura**
   p = parietal (adherent to the thoracic wall)
   v = visceral (adherent to the lung parenchyma)

10 **central tendon of the diaphragm**

11 **muscular crura of the diaphragm – opening for the oesophagus**

12 **arcuate ligament – opening for the aorta**

13 **pleural space i.e. b/n the pleural layers & below the lungs**
   (contains fluid - no air)

14 **opening in the central tendon for the IVC**

15 **pericardial space**

16 **intercostal muscles**
   e = external intercostals
   i = internal intercostals
   ii = innermost intercostals

17 **long thoracic a L&R**

18 **intercostal arteries (a) & Ns (n)**

(1 + 2 + 3 + 4)

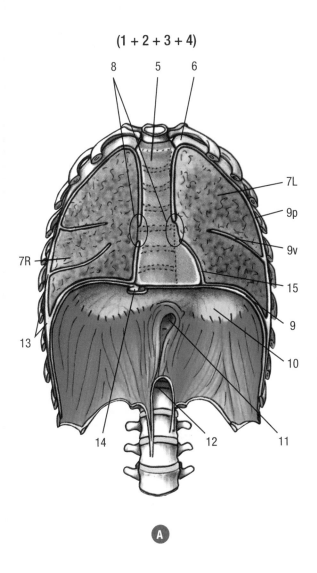

8   5   6

7L

9p

9v

7R

15

13

9

10

14   12   11

A

© A. L. Neill

195

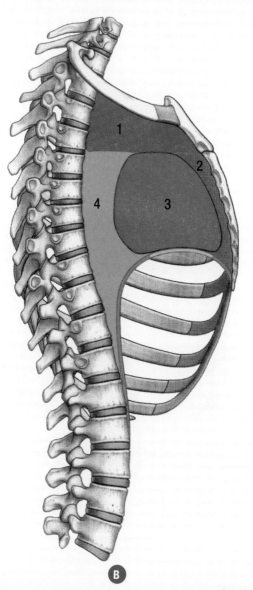

© A. L. Neill

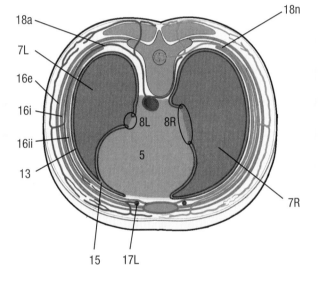

18a

18n

7L

16e

16i

16ii

13

8L

8R

5

7R

15

17L

C

Mouth AKA Oral cavity

Diagram of the normal oral cavity

1 **palate**
    h = hard / s = soft
2 **palatine arches**
    g = palatoglossal arch / p = palatopharyngeal arch
3 **palatine tonsil**
4 **oral part of the tongue = anterior 2/3**
5 **oral mucosa**
    b = buccal (on the side of the cheek)
    i = lingual (on the side of the tongue)
6 **back of the throat - oropharynx - posterior wall**
7 **mucosal folds / transverse & vertical**
8 **uvula - combination of mucosa & muscle**

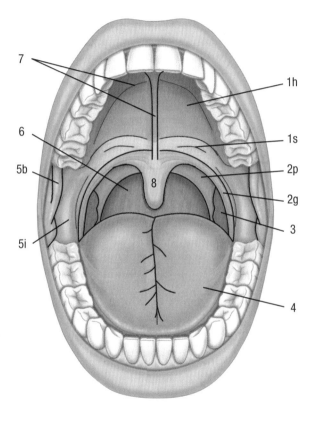

Muscles of Respiration

Diagram of the 1° & 2° muscles of respiration.

The major - **1° muscles of INSPIRATION are the ext. ICs , the interchondrial portion of the int. ICs & the diaphragm**, while those of **EXPIRATION are the int. ICs & the abdominal muscles**. In quiet respiration - the recoil of the elastic T & the weight of the ribs & muscles are generally sufficient.

The muscles keep the thoracic wall rigid & intact during respiration.

The arrows indicate the direction of contraction of the muscles (the diaphragm flattens out in contraction ↓ dome height ↑ thoracic diameter).

1   scalene mus. - ant. middle & post. (a, m & p)
2   sternocleidomastoid mu
3   ext. IC mu
4   int. IC mu
        i = interchondral section of the mu
5   innermost IC mu
6   external oblique mu
7   rectus abdominus mu
8   internal oblique mu
9   transversus abdominus mu
10 quadratus lumborum
11 diaphragm

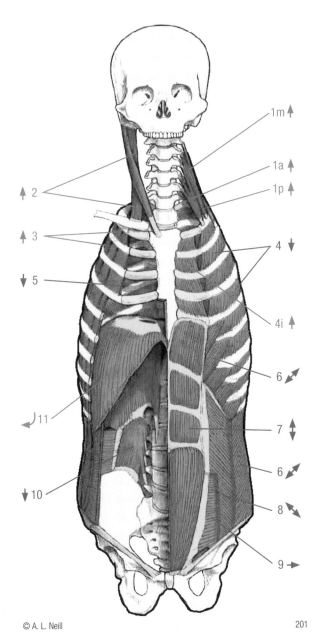

1m ↑
1a ↑
1p ↑
↑ 2
↑ 3
4 ↓
5 ↓
4i ↑
6 ↗↙
11
7 ↕
6 ↗↙
10 ↓
8 ↗↙
9 →

© A. L. Neill

Diaphragm

Anterior view of the diaphragm & posterior thoracic wall

The diaphragm in relaxation arches into the thoracic cavity & allows the rib cage to narrow; with contraction the muscles shorten causing it to flatten draw air in & & push out the rib cage diameter. Note the central tendon only moves up & down with respiratory movements, but the opening does not change - protecting the passage of the IVC. However the muscle crura wrap around the oesophagus & act as a physiological sphincter, preventing gastric reflux as abdominal pressure increases, in inspiration.

1 **trachea**

2 **common carotid a (L&R)**

3 **subclavian a**

4 **aorta**
   a = arch of the aorta
   d = descending aorta - t = thoracic part

5 **main bronchi AKA primary bronchi (L&R) - note R more vertical than the L which is pushed upwards due to the heart**

6 **diaphragm**
   c = arcuate lig
   m = muscular part - skeletal muscle
   t = tendinous section AKA central tendon of the diaphragm
   v = opening for the IVC

7 **oesophagus**

8 **brachiocephalic a**

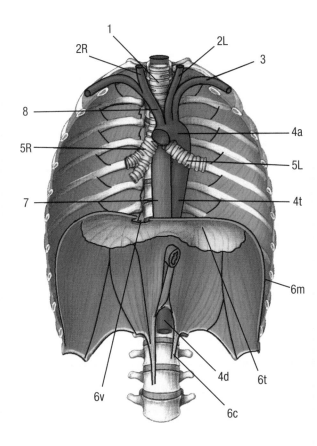

Diaphragm

Inferior view - looked at from below showing BS & NS

The BS of the diaphragm comes from below - phrenic arteries & veins, but the NS pierces the diaphragm from above - phrenic Ns.

In its relaxed state the diaphragm forms 2 domes, allowing the contents of the abdomen to push into the thorax. When activated the abdominal pressure is increased as the diaphragm flattens, increasing lung volume.

1   **Xiphisternum = Sternum + Xiphoid process**
2   **costal margin - cartilage**
3   **central tendon**
4   **rib - joining the costal margin**
5   **phrenic N = C 3,4,5 -   L = left & R = right**
6   **phrenic artery   L = left & R = right**
      a = lateral branch
      n = anterior branch
7   **aorta**
8   **Psoas muscle**
      a = major
      i = minor
9   **lumbar VB L4**
10 **crura (legs) of the diaphragm**
      L = left crus - inserts into VB L2
      R = right crus - longer - inserts into VB L3
11 **LP of the lumbar vertebrae**
12 **arcuate ligs - allowing the passage of structures from the thorax to the abdominal region w/o interfering with the diaphragmatic movements**
      a = lateral arcuate lig
      e = medial arcuate lig
13 **skeletal muscle of the diaphragmatic domes**
      L = left
      R = right - this dome is higher
14 **opening in the central tendon for the passage of the IVC**
15 **oesophagus passing b/n the crura of the diaphragm - physiological sphincter separating the stomach and lower oesophagus**

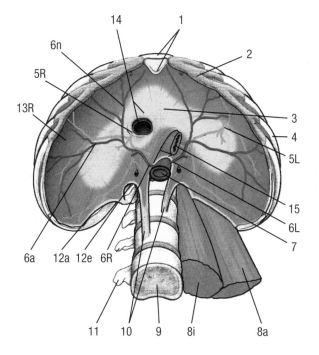

Nose & Nasal Cavity

A - lateral view

B - inferior view

The nose sits in the middle of the face. The cavity deep to the pyramidal structure is the nasal cavity, & the beginning of the RT. As well as moistening & streamlining the airflow the nose is responsible for olfaction AKA smelling.

Separated from the oral cavity (mouth) by the palate, they both open into the pharynx.

While the upper portion is boney the lower is fibrocartilgenous T.

Most bumps in the nose are due to the nasal bones. With time the fibro fatty T may harden & expand particularly in the male making the external structure much larger - Rhinophyma.

1   **Frontal bone**
2   **Nasal bones**
3   **lateral cartilages**
4   **alar cartilages - major**
5   **alar cartilages - minor -with adherent skin**
6   **fibro fatty T**
7   **Maxilla - frontal process**
8   **septal cartilage**
9   **nostril AKA nare**

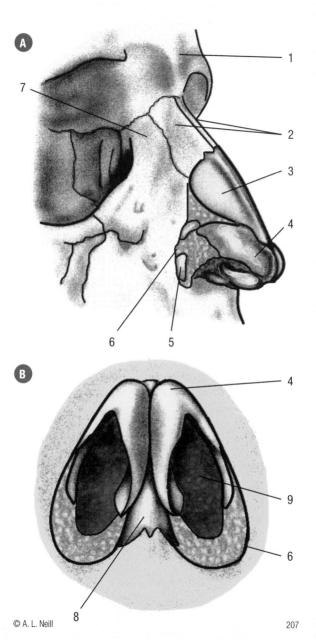

Nose – in situ

Lateral, Medial

The nose consists of the nasal cavity & the surrounding structures around that cavity. These are made up of many contributing bones similar to the paranasal sinuses, & other structures such as cartilages.

1 **Frontal bone, 1s = Frontal sinus**
2 **Nasal bone**
3 **Nasal cartilages – 3L= lateral cartilage**
   3A = alar cartilage, 3S= septal cartilage
4 **Nostril = nare = nasal opening**
5 **Lips**
6 **Maxilla – with tooth embedded**
7 **Palatine bone (making up the hard palate)**
   7i = incisive canal
8 **Inferior concha**
9 **Sphenoid bone**
   9L= lateral pterygoid plate 9s = Sphenoid sinus
10 **Ethmoid bone**
   10c = cribiform plate, 10m = medial concha
   10p = perpendicular plate, 10s = superior concha
11 **Sphenopalatine foramen**
12 **Lacrimal bone**
13 **Vomer**

contribution of the Frontal bone
contribution of the Sphenoid
contribution of the Maxilla
contribution of the Ethmoid bone
inferior nasal concha (is its own bone)
Vomer
Nasal bone
Lacrimal bone
contribution of the Palatine bone
cartilages

© A. L. Neill

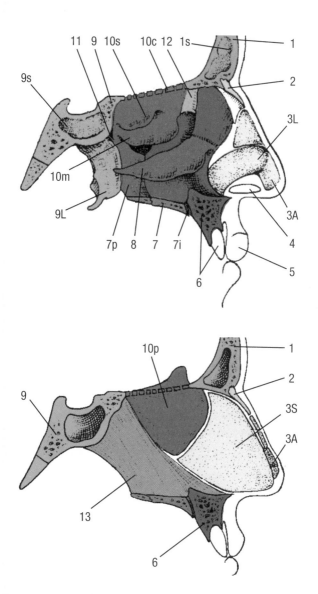

Nose & Nasal Cavity - Blood Supply

A - lateral view

B - medial view

The nose is supplied by several facial art. which aa extensively in the septum & at the tip of the nose.

The nasal cartilages continue to grow throughout life, & need a strong BS as cartilage does not have any BVs w/n the T. The nose is prone to ly & copious bleeding. Repeated nose bleeds may be a sign of more serious pathology e.g. hypertension.

1 **ethmoidal a**
> **a = anterior / p = posterior**

2 **spheno-palantine a**
> **L = lateral br**
> **s = septal br**

3 **terminal br of greater palatine a**

4 **lat. nasal a**
> **a = alar br**
> **L = labial br**

5 **alar cartilages**

6 **upper lip**

7 **septal br of 1a**

8 **septal br of 1p**

9 **Little's area anastomoses from 3 major BVs**
> **2s + 7 + 8 - area where most nose-bleeds originate (epistaxis)**

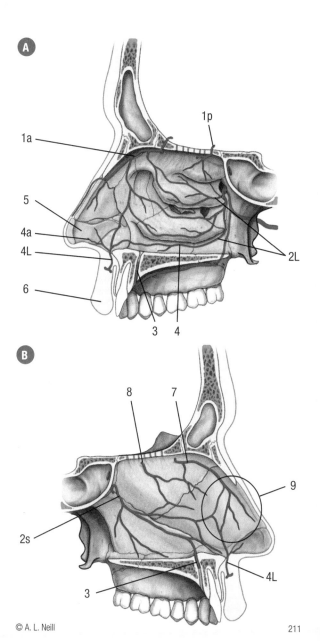

Nose & Nasal Cavity - Nerve Supply

A - lateral view

B - medial view

The nose is supplied by branches of the CN V1, 2

It also has a special NS from CN 1 - the Olfactory N.

1   **CN I - Olfactory N branches pierce cribriform plate of the Ethmoid b & emerge through the nasal mucosa**

2   **ethmoidal N**
>   **a = anterior / p = posterior**
>   **s = septal (from V1)**

3   **internal nasal br of V2 (infraorbital N) (from V2)**

4   **br of ant. superior alveolar N (from V2)**

5   **posterior lateral N - s = superior br**
>   **- i = inferior br   (from V2)**

6   **alar cartilages**

7   **nasopalatine N (from V2)**

8   **septal cartilage**

9   **hard palate = Palatine b**

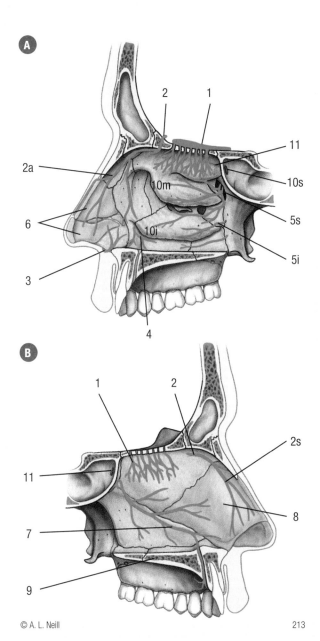

Nasal Mucosa junctional region

Histology of the junction b/n the normal respiratory lining (R) & the specialized olfactory mucosa (O)

Specialized olfactory glands & N endings represent in the specialized area. These are replaced by the normal PSCCE & respiratory glands of the URT.

1. **non- motile cilia - similar to long mv of the supportive cells**
2. **pore of Bowman's gland AKA olfactory glands**
3. **N process**
4. **olfactory glands AKA Bowman's glands**
5. **basal cell**
6. **BM**
7. **olfactory N processes which extend processes opening onto the surface**
8. **capillary**
9. **venule**
10. **arteriole**
11. **lamina propria**
12. **cilia**
13. **goblet cell**

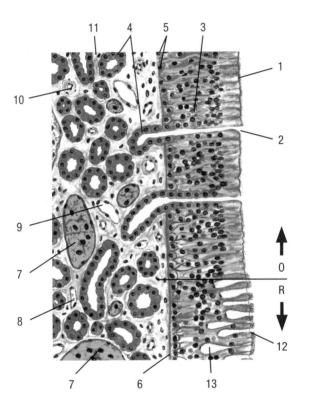

Olfactory Mucosa AKA Nasal Mucosa

Diagram of the microanatomy of the olfactory mucosal lining upper nasal cavity

Sensitive N endings cover the ciliated mucosal surface and coalesce to form the Olfactory N CN I

1 non- motile cilia - AKA stereocilia, long mv.
2 supportive cells AKA sustenacular cells
3 non-myelinated axons
4 olfactory glands AKA Bowman's glands
5 basal cell
6 olfactory sensory cell
7 dendritic process opening onto the surface
8 sensory processes of the olfactory cells - neurocilia
9 pore of the glands - moistens the mucosal surface
10 fusion of axon forming CN I
11 junctional complex

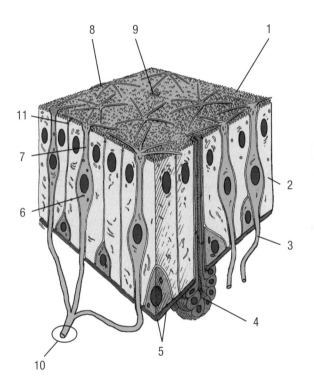

Pharynx - Divisions of

Diagram of the normal pharynx - sagittal view

The pharynx is the passage connecting the nasal & oral cavities. It has 3 divisions ending at the beginning of the oesophagus.

A = nasopharynx

B = oropharynx

C = laryngeal pharynx

A + B + C = pharynx

1   nasal cavity
2   palate
3   oral cavity
4   Mandible (lower jaw)
5   tongue
6   epiglottis
7   thyroid cart.
8   cricoid cart.
9   trachea
10 larynx
11 Eustachian tube opening
12 oesophagus

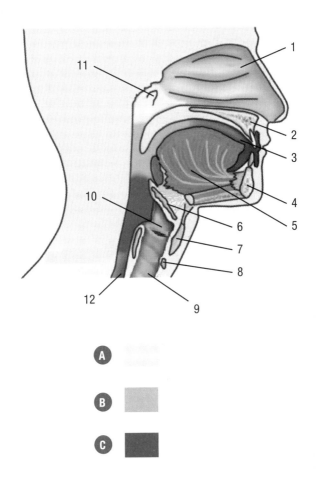

Pharynx - Divisions of

Posterior – schematic intact

Posterior – divided constrictor muscles

A - NASO-PHARYNX

B - ORO-PHARYNX

C - LARYNGO-PHARYNX

A + B + C - Pharynx

The pharynx (main part of the throat) is at the back of the mouth – 12cm (5 ins) long. It extends down the neck in the shape of an inverted cone connecting the mouth with the oesophagus. Elevating the soft palate closes the nasopharynx. This stops food coming out of the nose. Sneezing occurs when this closure becomes uncoordinated.

1 Skull
2 Adenoid tonsil
3 Soft palate
4 Phayngeal constrictors i = inf /m = middle/ s = superior
5 Epiglottis
6 laryngeal inlet
7 Cricoid cartilage
8 Oesophageal mucosa – continuous with oral mucosa
9 Oesophagus
10 Piriform fossa and opening to oesophagus
11 Oral mucosa – continues throughout the pharynx
12 Tonsil
13 Uvula
14 Orophayngeal isthmus
15 Palato-pharyngeal fold
16 Nasal choane = turbinates
17 Nasal septum
18 Thyroid gland
19 Parathyroid glands
20 Tracheal cartilage
21 Hyoid

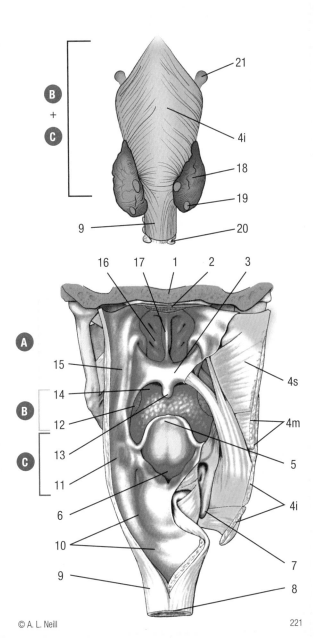

Pharynx - connections b/n divisions

Diagram of the normal pharynx - lateroposterior view

The pharynx is the passage connecting the nasal & oral cavities.
It has 3 divisions & ends at the beginning of the oesophagus.

A = nasopharynx
B = oropharynx
C = pharynx

Except for tensor veli palatini m (9); all muscles are innervated by the Vagus N - pharyngeal branch.

1   **Eustachian tube**
2   **levator veli palatini m**
3   **inf. turbinate b**
4   **palatine tonsil**
5   **muscularis uvulae m**
6   **palateopharyngeus m**
7   **superior pharyngeal constrictor m**
8   **pterygoid hamulus**
9   **tensor veli palatini m (CNV3 - mandibular N)***
10 **tongue**

Asking a patient to say AHHHH - should cause the palate to lift evenly (NAD) due to these muscles (5,6), but if there is any malfunction of the Vagus N (pharyngeal branch) then the uvula will be seen to move towards the healthy side (H), & the opening in the throat appears uneven. The patient will also have an ineffective long bovine cough, & may have sleep apnea. More details in **the A to Z of the Brain & Cranial Nerves**

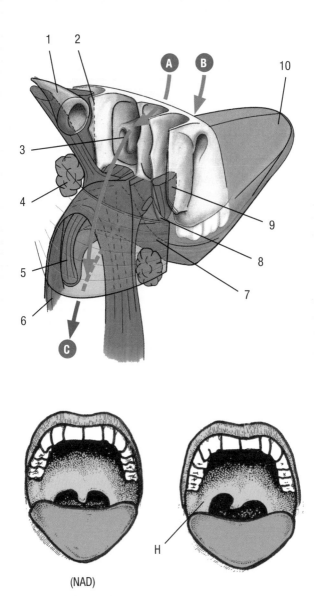

(NAD)

© A. L. Neill

Pleura - Parietal boundaries

Diagram of the extent of the parietal pleura

The parietal pleura is very sensitive to pain. Its NS comes from general somatic Ns, which supply the overlying muscles. The visceral pleura has a NS which comes from the visceral Ns, so it is relatively insensitive to pain.

1 **cervical pleura - comes above the first rib**
2 **opening for the pulmonary vessels**
3 **costal part of the pleura**
4 **pulmonary lig**
5 **diaphragmatic part**
6 **pleural extension - lies below the lung by ~2 - 4cm which changes with breathing**

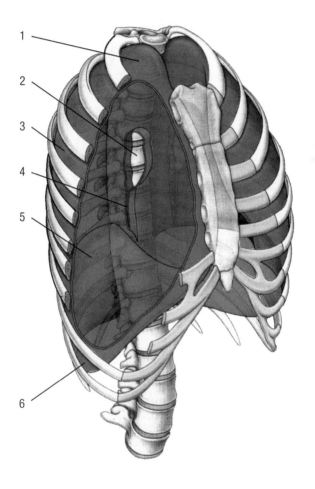

Open Pneumothorax

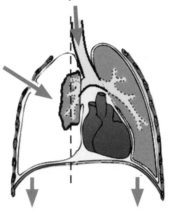

Tension Pneumothorax

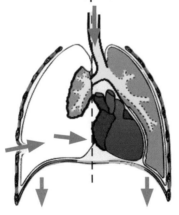

Open pneumothorax air may escape with each breath, but in the tension pneumothorax progressive inspirations, are trapped in the thorax and progressively move the mediastinal structures towards the closed side.

expiration

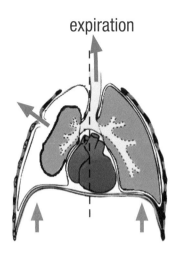

expiration

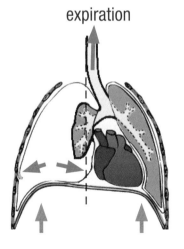

Sinuses AKA Parasinuses

Coronal view looked at from the front

The paranasal sinuses are generally the "sinuses" referred to when discussing sinus pain etc - they are the air filled spaces which empty into the nasal cavity. They may swell, become infected & fill with fluid, causing pain & pathology. A number of bones contribute to these spaces, as indicated.

1   **cranial vault (ACF at this point)**
2   **ethmoid air cells**
3   **maxillary sinus**
4   **nasal cavity**
5   **boney palate = hard palate**
6   **inferior meatus (opening)**
6A **inferior concha (turbinate)**
7   **middle meatus**
7A **middle concha (turbinate)**
8   **superior meatus**
8A **superior concha (turbinate)**
9   **orbit / orbital fossa**
10 **frontal sunis**
11 **sphenoid sinus**

▮ Contribution of the Frontal bone
▮ Contribution of the Zygoma
▮ **Contribution of the Maxilla**
▮ Contribution of the Ethmoid bone
▮ Inferior Nasal concha (is its own bone)
▮ **Vomer**

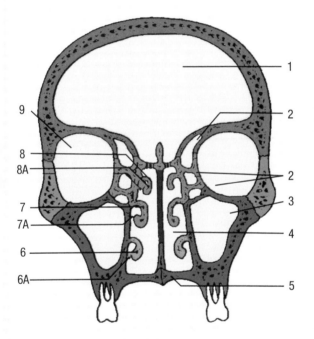

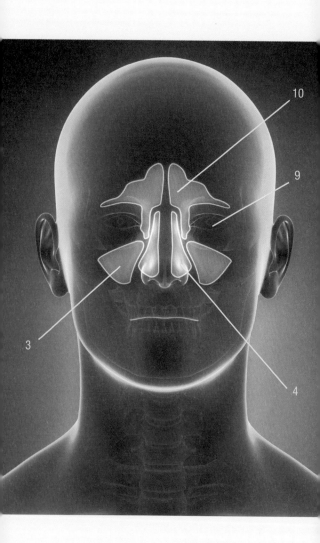

10

9

3

4

© A. L. Neill

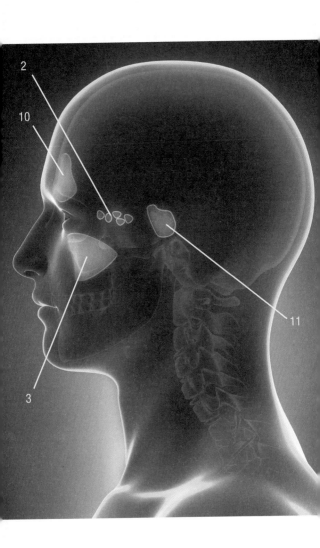

Sinuses AKA Paranasal sinuses

A - anterior view of nasal in the skull

B - sagittal view - looking into the centre of the skull

Air filled spaces- sinuses form in the skull to lighten it. They are lined with mucous secreting respiratory epithelium & drain into the nasal cavity. Increased secretions as an inflammatory or immune reactions result in fluid filled cavities which may be painful - sinusitis. Any blockage to the drainage due to swollen or congested noses also cause pain - sinusitis. The interconnections & extent of the sinuses vary considerably. Tooth abscesses, eye infections & other related infections in the area may spread to the sinuses. Note the proximity to the pituitary gland.

1 **frontal sinus - if blocked often produce "sinus headaches"**

2 **ethmoid sinuses - often multiple small air cells which easily block**

3 **maxillary sinus - maybe affected by dental infections of the teeth &/or gums**

4 **sphenoid sinus**

5 **pituitary gland - note proximity to 4**

6 **nasal conchae -**

> **i = inferior - a separate bone in the nose often enlarged & may block the sinus drainage**
>
> **m = middle**
>
> **s = superior**

7 **nasal septum**

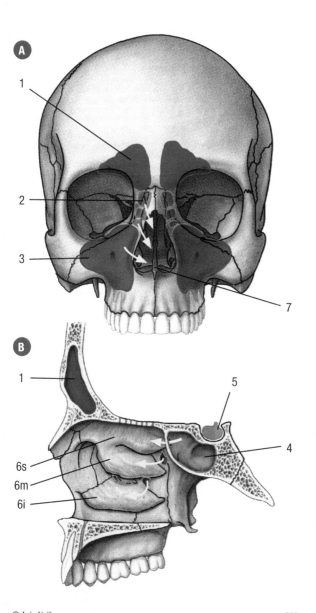

Sinuses AKA Parasinuses

A - Coronal - Frontal, looking onto the nose

B - Transverse - looking across the nasal cavity

Radiology

The paranasal sinuses are generally the "sinuses" referred to when discussing sinus pain etc - they are the air filled spaces which empty into the nasal cavity and communicate with each other with many variations.

They may become involved in the spread of infection and cancer throughout the Head, Face and Cranial cavities.

1   Cranial vault (ACF at this point)
2   Frontal sinus
3   Ethmoid sinuses / spaces
   a = ant. cells / p = post. cells
   i = infundibulum leading to the maxillary sinus (5)
   pp = perpendicular plate
   u = uncinate process
4   floor of the orbital cavity –
   c = infra-orbital canal
   s = additional sinus in the floor of the orbit – varies
5   Maxillary sinus
6   Nasal conchae
   i = inf. nasal concha
   m = middle nasal concha
   s = superior nasal concha
7   Vomer
8   Nasal septum
   t = tubercle i.e. some septi have swellings & overgrowths as well as deviations interfering with breathing
9   Middle nasal meatus (opening)
10 Orbital cavity showing eyeball and peri-orbital fat
11 Crista galli – this one pneumatised (air filled) – varies
12 Lateral rectus
13 Sphenoid sinuses

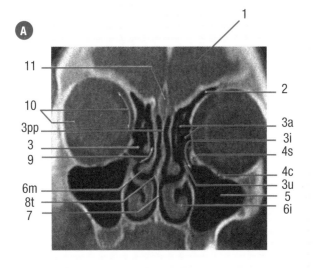

A

1

11

10

3pp

3

9

6m

8t

7

2

3a

3i

4s

4c

3u

5

6i

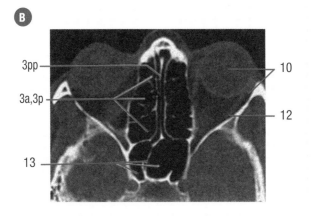

B

3pp

3a,3p

13

10

12

Thoracic Linings + Spaces

Diagram of the membranes lining the sections of the thoracic cavity - pleural & pericardial - anterolateral

The parietal pleura is very sensitive to pain, as is the fibrous pericardium, which it fuses with along the mediastinal walls & at the base. These membranes keep the compartments in the thorax separate & in position. The pleura must be intact & are essential for respiration but the pericardium is not essential to the heart.

1 **pleural spaces L & R**
    come above rib 1 in the neck
    bound by the inner thoracic walls laterally
    bound by the superior surface of the diaphragm inferiorly

2 **mediastinum - medial boundary of the pleural spaces**

3 **Manubrium**

4 **sternal angle**

5 **Sternum**

6 **Xiphoid**

7 **rib 7**

8 **diaphragm inf. surface**

9 **pleural cavity extends below & medial to the lung T & contains fluid**

10 **fibrous pericardium, fuses with the parietal pleura medially**

11 **fibrous pericardium fuses with the central tendon inferiorly**

12 **thoracic outlets i = inf. / s = sup.**

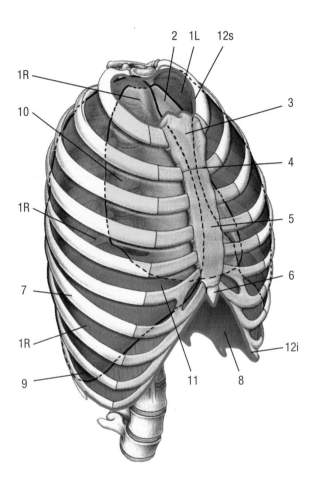

Thoracic Outlets

A - *superior thoracic outlet AKA thoracic inlet AKA superior thoracic aperture AKA thoracic outlet*

B - *inferior thoracic outlet AKA inferior thoracic aperture AKA thoracic outlet*

C - *brachial plexus & brachial BVs with arm raised & not raised*

D - *pectoral girdle - superior view*

The thoracic outlets are boundaries for the thorax, separating it from the root of the neck superiorly & the abdomen inferiorly. Vital structures pass though both. If obstructed the BS & function of the UL may be compromised superiorly - Thoracic Outlet Syndrome & the BS to the GIT & LLs inferiorly.

1 **rib 1**
2 **rib 2**
3 **T1**
4 **true ribs 1-7 - articulate with the Sternum directly**
5 **false ribs 8-10 - articulate anteriorly via costal cartilage**
6 **floating ribs 11-12 - do not articulate anteriorly**
7 **L1**
8 **costal cartilage**
9 **L3**
10 **intercostal space**
11 **thoracic outlets**
    i = inferior
    s = superior
12 **Clavicle**
13 **scalene muscles**
    a = anterior
    m = middle
14 **brachial plexus (BP) - anterior SN roots**
15 **subclavian BVs & Ns from the BP - reforming**
16 **brachial BVs & Ns from the BP - PNs supplying the UL**
17 **Scapula**
    a = acromial process (acromium)
    c = coracoid process
18 **Humerus**
19 **Pectoralis minor mu**

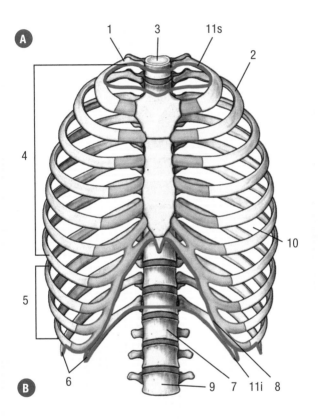

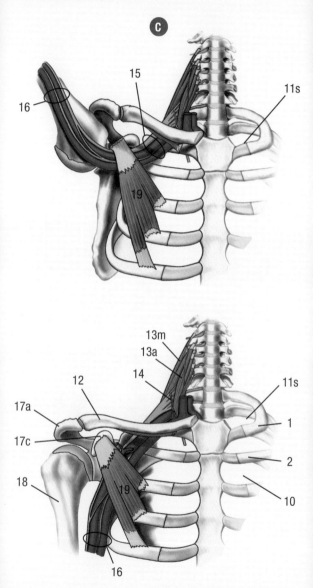

© A. L. Neill

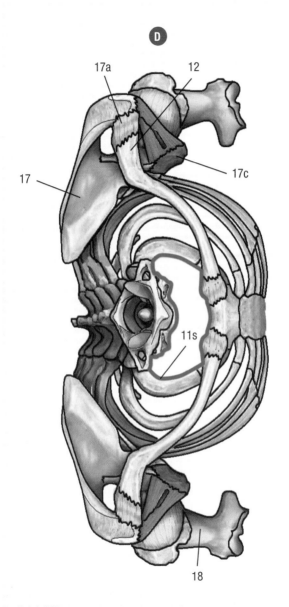

17a

12

17

17c

11s

18

© A. L. Neill

Thoracic Wall - anterior

View of the interior of the anterior chest wall - Parietal pleura removed

1 internal IC m ..

2 innermost IC m

3 transverse thoracis m..

4 Xiphoid process (hyaline cartilage which ossifies with age)

5 external oblique

      a = aponeurotic part

      m = muscular part

6 diaphragm m ..

7 IC space

8 IC vein art. & N (sup. → inf.)

      AKA IC neurovascular bundle

9 Clavicle b

10 first rib -

      costal cartilage, bone, cut bone (medial → lateral)

11 scalene muscles

12 long thoracic a&v

13 Manubrium b

14 Sternum b

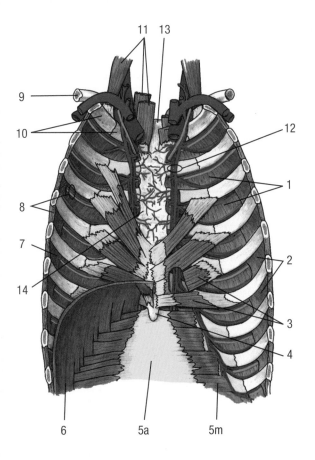

Thoracic wall – Posterior

Anterior view of the internal surface of the posterior thoracic wall - heart, lungs, lymphatic & veins removed

The thoracic aorta lies in the posterior mediastinum which can be further divided into the ascending aorta, the arch of the aorta and the descending aorta (above the diaphragm)

It is highly segmental & branches supply: the ribs, contents of the IC spaces, the oesophagus, the trachea & bronchi, the lung pleural tissues and the pericardium.

1 **oesophagus**
2 **L common carotid & subclavian a**
3 **arch of the aorta**
4 **carina (point of bifurcation of the trachea)**
5 **brs arising from the aorta**
      b = bronchial
      o = oesophageal
      p = pericardial
6 **diaphragm – central ligament**
7 **opening for the IVC**
8 **IC a – part of the IC neurovascular bundle**
9 **R main bronchus (note more vertical than the L)**
10 **tracheal & R bronchial a**
11 **trachea**
12 **R brachiocephalic a**
13 **innermost IC m**
14 **-internal IC m**
15 **first rib**

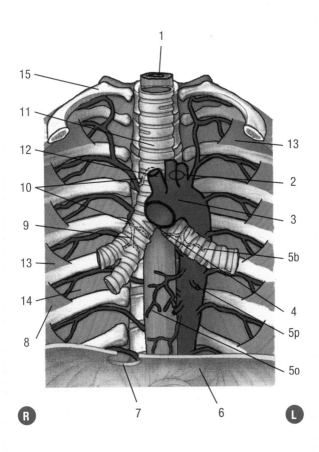

R

L

Thoracic wall – Posterior

Interior view of the posterior thoracic wall
Lymphatic drainage - Aorta & Azygos system removed

The lymphatics drain each ICS & form large ducts to empty at the intersection of the jugular & subclavian veins on the L&R. While the drainage is symmetrical in the thoracic region this is not the case in other areas.

1 **duct emptying into junction of L subclavian & jugular v**
2 **L subclavian v**
3 **L 2nd & 3rd ribs**
4 **thoracic duct = L lymphatic duct**
5 **LNs**
6 **IC lymphatic vessels**
7 **L lumbar lymphatic trunk**
8 **IVC**
9 **cisterna chyli**
10 **R thoracic duct = R lymphatic duct**
11 **SVC**
12 **duct emptying into R subclavian & jugular v**
13 **R jugular v**
14 **oesophagus**
15 **L common carotid art & L jugular v**

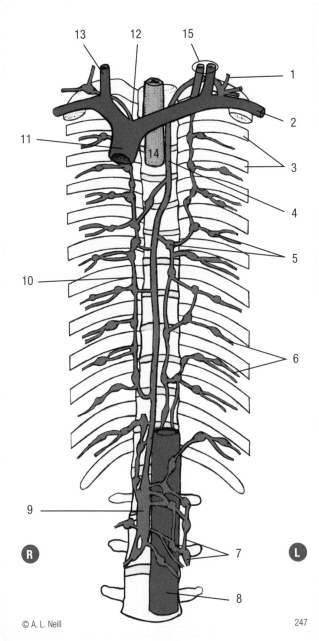

R

L

© A. L. Neill

Thoracic wall – Posterior

Interior view of the posterior thoracic wall - NS

1 vagus N
2 cervical sympathetic ganglion
3 3rd ICN
4 sympathetic chain
5 cardiac N plexus
6 L greater splanchnic N
7 anterior vagal trunk
8 coeliac N plexus & ganglia
9 oesophageal N plexus
10 brachial N plexus
11 trachea
12 oesophagus

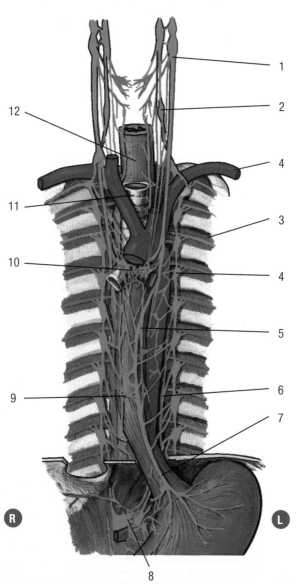

R

L

© A. L. Neill

Thoracic wall – Posterior

Interior view of the posterior thoracic wall - venous drainage

A lateral

B posterior

1 **SVC**
2 **IVC**
3 **IC v - a accessory IC v**
4 **azygous v**
5 **hemi-azygous v**
6 **accessory hemi-azygous v**
7 **L brachiocephalic v**
8 **Scapula**
9 **long thoracic v AKA internal thoracic v**

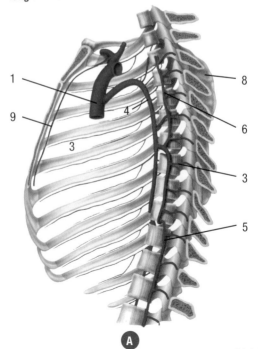

A

© A. L. Neill

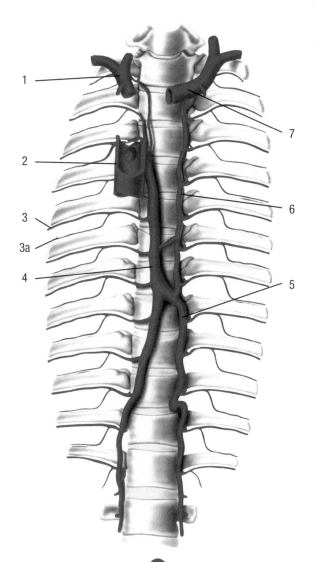

1

2

3

3a

4

7

6

5

© A. L. Neill

B

Thoracic wall - Blood Supply

A - posterior view of body BVs VC & SC removed - posterior ribs of the L side removed

The segmental nature of the BS of the thorax is contrasted with the less organized BS of the abdomen, pelvis and head & neck.

1 **aorta**

    t = thoracic aorta

2 **SVC**

3 **IVC**

4 **azygos v h = hemi-azygos v**

5 **IC neurovascular bundle = intercostal vein, artery & nerve from superior to inferior the components run under the costal groove in the order of VAN**

    c = collateral br - spread over the IC space to innervate the structures in the space (variable)

6 **IC muscles of the thoracic wall change the shape of the wall & alter the volume of the thorax**

    e = external IC - outermost muscles, deficient ant., bring the ribs up & out, ↑ thoracic volume

    i = internal IC - muscle fibres run in the opposite direction - ↓ thorax

    ii = innermost IC - muscles fibres vary in direction mainly AP or along with internal ICs assist ↓ thorax - deficient ant. & post. (AKA intercostal intimi)

    f = fascia in the anterior

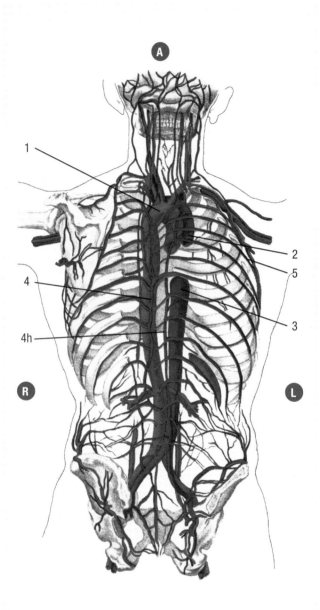

B - BS & NS of a typical IC space showing perforating branches

C - anterolateral view of the chest wall - with segment demonstrating relationship b/n BVs, muscles & Ns (lymphatics not shown)

7 **SC**
8 **posterior perforating br of IC bundle (a, v & N)**
9 **lateral perforating br of IC bundle (a, v & N)**
10 **anterior perforating br of IC bundle (a, v & N)**
11 **internal thoracic art & vein AKA ant. mammary a &v**
12 **costal groove - this protects the IC bundle**
13 **diaphragm**

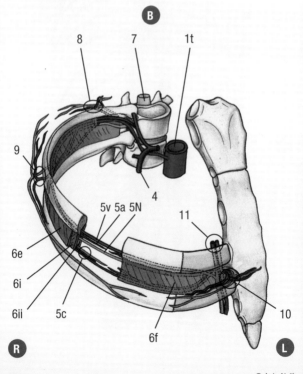

© A. L. Neill

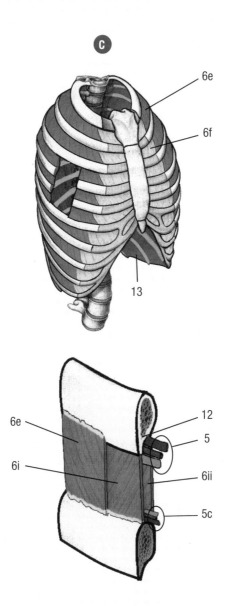

6e

6f

13

6e

6i

12

5

6ii

5c

© A. L. Neill

Thoracic walls - Nerve Supply

A - posterio-lateral view of thoracic SC & VC to show origins of SNs & the IC Ns

The segmental nature of the NS of the thorax is contrasted with that of the appendicular skeleton and pelvic NS.

B - posterior view of the skeleton with SP of the VC removed to show origins of the SNs

C - posterior view of the axial skeleton to show regional differences in the VC and boney protection of Ns

The thoracic Ns are protected by bone for most of their pathway, in particular note the down-pointing thoracic SPs. The thoracic SNs remain segmental & do not form ansae unlike the various N plexi which supply the appendicular skeleton.

1 **IC Ns**

2 **Ns of the BP**

3 **Ns of the LP**

4 **Ns of the SP**

5 **Sciatic N**

6 **SC**

7 **SP of thoracic vertebra**

8 **costovertebral jt b/n TP & rib**

9 **cervical vertebrae, long bifid SPs become more like typical thoracic vertebrae**

10 **lumbar vertebrae, note exposure b/n the vertebrae, which allows for additional mobility but also the ↑ risk of N compression with movement**

11 **Sacrum**

12 **T12 - note the transition with progression through the thorax towards horizontal SPs. This vertebra resembles a lumbar VB**

13 **Scapula - removed on R to show the rib cage**

14 **Clavicle - removed on R to show the rib cage**

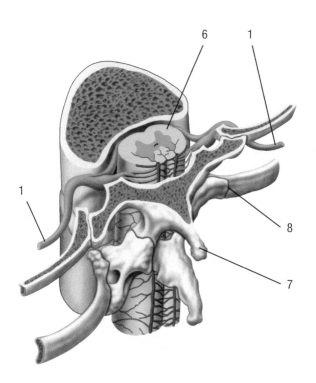

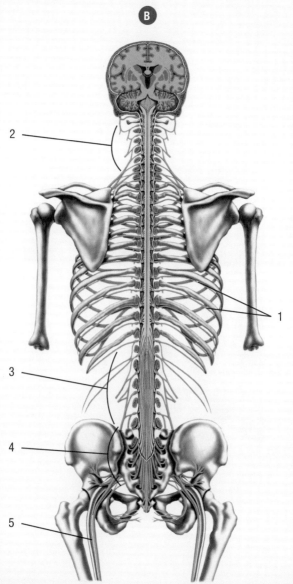

2

1

3

4

5

© A. L. Neill

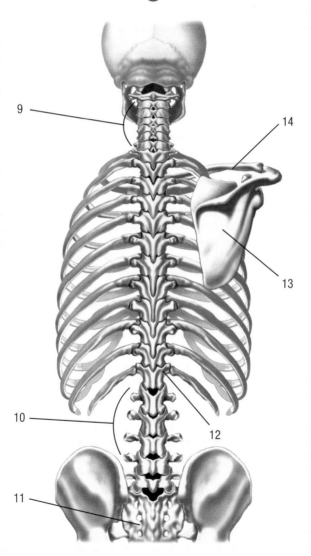

Thoracic Segment - BS & muscles

Diagram of the arterial supply of thoracic segments - transverse

A - anterior

P - posterior

Each thoracic segment is supplied by branches of the thoracic aorta. These give off a posterior branch to supply the muscles of the back & at the mid-axially line a lateral cutaneous branch. The vessels travel on the inf. margin of their associated rib b/n the innermost & internal IC muscles with the IC veins & Ns. The long thoracic artery (AKA mammary a AKA internal thoracic a) give off ant. branches which anastomose with the arteries of the posterior ICs. A thoracic segment is the space b/n the ribs - IC space 4 is b/n ribs 3 & 4.

1 **thoracic aorta**

2 **rib**

3 **IC N**

4 **long thoracic a AKA mammary a**
      a = anterior perforating br

5 **subcut fat -**

6 **lateral perforating br of IC N which also has an ant. br (a) & post br (p)**

7 **sympathetic ganglion**

8 **L post. a (from aorta) - note travels straight back**
      a = sup. br which becomes SC.
      d = deep posterior

9 **R post a (from the thoracic aorta - across the VC)**

10 **superior epigastric a**

11 **anterior perforating br of the IC N**
      a =ant. br
      L = lat. br

12 **4th IC space b/n ribs 3 & 4**

13 **thoracic cavity**

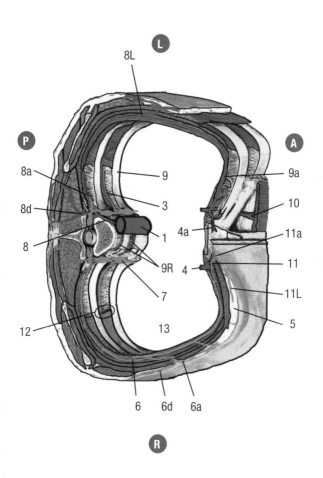

L

P

A

8L

8a

9

9a

8d

3

8

10

4a

1

11a

9R

4

11

7

11L

12

5

13

6

6d

6a

R

Thoracic Segment - Nerve Supply

Diagram of the innervation of each thoracic segment - transverse

A - anterior

P - posterior

Each thoracic segment of the SC has a dorsal (pure sensory) & ventral root (pure motor) which combines to form the mixed spinal N. The SN then splits into a ventral ramus (branch) & dorsal ramus which supply the intercostal segment (space b/n the 2 ribs) & back muscles respectively. In the lower thorax, the medial branch is shorter so that the dorsal branch supplies most of the sensation and motor activity of the muscles & skin below the ribs as well as the back muscles.

1   **spinal cord (SC)**
2   **SN**
        d = dorsal root
        g = dorsal root ganglion
        v = ventral root
3   **sympathetic chain**
4   **ventral branch of SN = intercostal N**
        a = anterior perforating br
        L = lateral perforating br
5   **dorsal branch of SN - supplies the back muscles segmentally -**
6   **Scapula**
7   **spinal canal**
8   **VB**
9   **erector spinae - major muscle group of the back**

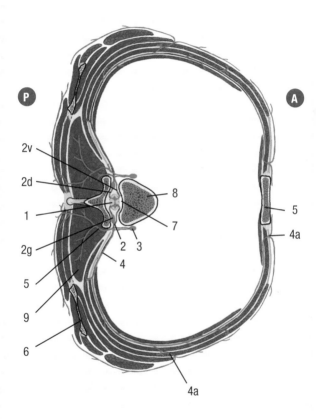

P

A

2v

2d

1

2g

5

9

6

8

7

3

2

4

5

4a

4a

Throat – overview

Lateral view – with tissues cut away to show their relationships.

A - nasal cavity

B - oral cavity

C - nasaopharynx

D - oropharynx

E - laryngopharnyx

C + D + E - pharynx

The throat is the passage through which everything must pass: air, food & liquids. It is the junction point of the oral and nasal passages, separating the air from the solid material via the epiglottis. It also connects with the ears via their drainage channels the Eustachian tubes. The Pharnyx – a muscular tube from the base of the skull to the oesophagus is its main component.

1 **Hard palate**
2 **Glossopharyngeal N**
3 **Epiglottis**
4 **Cricoid cartilage = Adams apple**
5 **Trachea = air passage**
6 **Oesophagus = food passage**
7 **Eustachain tube = auditory tube**
8 **Soft Palate**

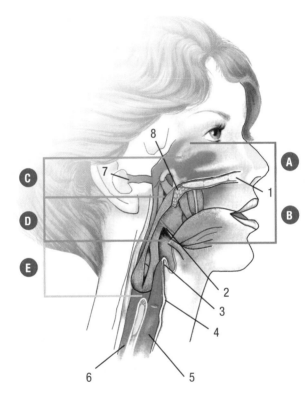

Throat - muscles

Posterior overview of a coronal section of the muscles of the pharynx - back of the throat

The tone of the muscles in this area may change & slacken leading to sleep apnea, snoring &/or dysphagia.

Other Ts notably the tonsils can enlarge in infections and block the airways.

Yawning involves muscles 9 + 10 & the medial pterygoid (not shown)

1 **hard palate**

2 **Eustachian tube**

3 **Ethmoid b**

4 **Vomer b - separates the nostrils**

5 **palatine tonsilar T (adenoids)- may enlarge & obstruct the nasal passage in Ins / much larger in children**

6 **inferior concha - a separate bone in the nasal cavity - the other conchae are projections of the Ethmoid b**

7 **tongue - floor of the mouth & pharynx - moving posteriorly blocks the airway (cf sleep apnea)**

8 **palatopharyngeus & deeper is the superior pharyngeal m**

9 **muscularis uvulae m**

10 **levator tensor palatini + salpingopharngeus m**

11 **digastric & deeper is tensor veli palatini m**

*9 + 10 open the pharynx & the Eustachian tubes
8 + 11 lift & narrow the pharynx (cf swallowing)

* for more details on individual muscles see *the A to Z of the Head & Neck* - muscle section

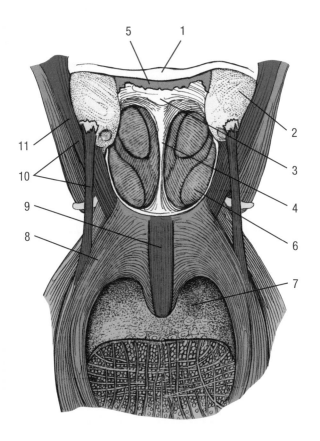

Differences between Normal (A), Bacterial (B) & Viral (V) Throat infections & Tonsillitis

The appearances of the throat with tonsillitis vary with the causative agent.

	A - normal	B - bacterial	C- viral
1 - tonsil	pink / red	red swollen with white or cream spots ++++	red swollen ++
2 - uvula	pink / red / soft	red / swollen ++	red / swollen ±
3 - throat	pink / shiny	sore / red ++++	sore / red ++
4 - tongue	pink / uncoated	enlarged / coated white or grey unusual texture "feels funny"	red / enlarged / uncoated

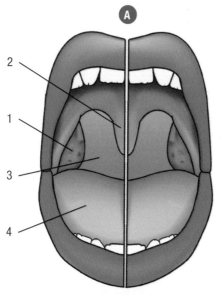

A

268

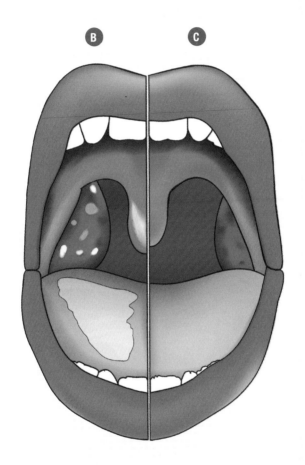

Tonsils – in situ

Lateral view - with tissues cut away to show their relationships

Mouth of a child

The tonsils form a defense ring around air and food pathways. Even though they play a role in the defense of substances passing through – in infected states – tonsilitis -they swell and compromise access of air and food to the body.

1 **Nasopharynx**
2 **Hard Palate**
3 **Oropharynx**
4 **Tongue**
5 **Lingual tonsil – on the root of the tongue**
6 **Epiglottis – Vallecula**
7 **Palatine tonsil**
8 **Pharyngeal folds/arches – for funnelling food into the oesophagus**
9 **Adenoids = Pharyngeal tonsils**
10 **Nasopharynx**

As the mouth – jaw increases in size so does the pharynx – and swollen tonsils are not as obstructive to food and air

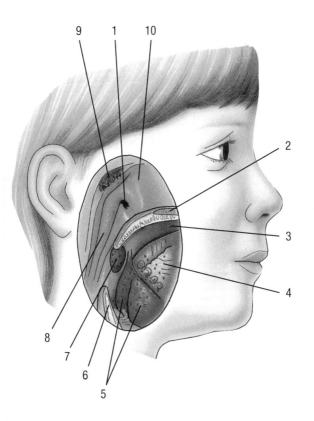

Trachea - in situ

Macroscopic view of the relationship b/n the trachea, oesophagus, & the thyroid gland at 2 levels C6 & T1

1   thyroid parenchyma with CT septa
2   tracheal fascia
3   isthmus - -showing cut surface & superior edge
4   superior thyroid a & v
5   anterior surface of the L lobe
6   middle cervical fascia = pretracheal fascia
7   superior pole of R thyroid lobe
8   internal jugular v
9   common carotid a
10 prevertebral fascia
11 trachea
12 T1 vertebral body
13 oesophagus
14 recurrent laryngeal N L&R
15 L Vagus N
16 Ns of the Brachial Plexus

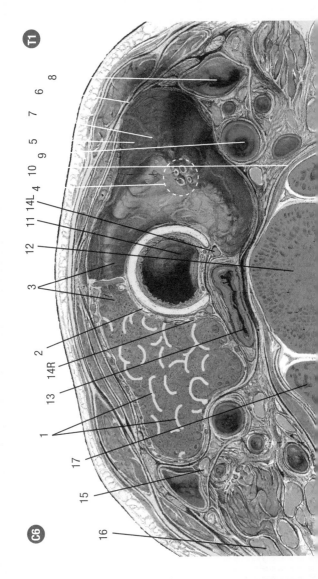

T1

8
6
7
5
9
4
10
14L
11 14
12
3
2
14R
13
1
17
15

C6

16

© A. L. Neill

273

Tracheal wall

A - LP H&E trachea

B - HP H&E trachea

The lining of the trachea is a thick folded mucosa. Its main function is to ensure the air is dust free, warm & moist. Hence the numerous seromucosal glands & PSCCE lumenal lining. The lumen is maintained by cartilaginous rings. Posteriorly the connecting smooth muscle allows for the oesophagus to expand with food ingestion, w/o compromising the tracheal lumen.

1   demilune of the seromucous gld
2   serous gld
3   BM
4   PSCCE - this T changes with irritation to become truly stratified
5   cilia lining the trachea, these structures are lost with metaplasia of the epithelium
6   goblet cells
7   nuclear rows - note this is a simple epithelium - i.e. all the cells touch the BM & only the nuclei are multilayered
8   pulmonary v
9   duct
10 pulmonary a
11 hyaline cartilage - part of the tracheal ring
12 perichondrium
13 smooth muscle - posterior wall of the trachea
14 adventitia
15 adipose T
16 mucosal folds - lamina propria
17 elastic fibres
18 Ns

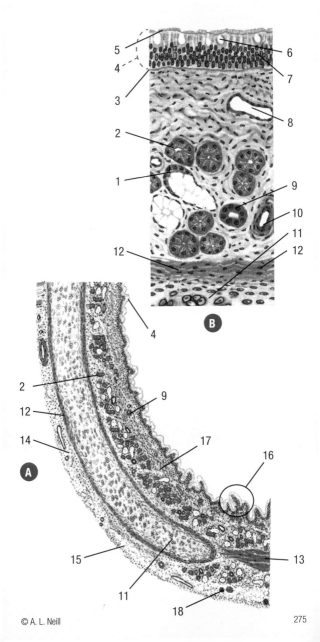

© A. L. Neill

Additional Images

Quizzes